OPHTHALMIC NURSING

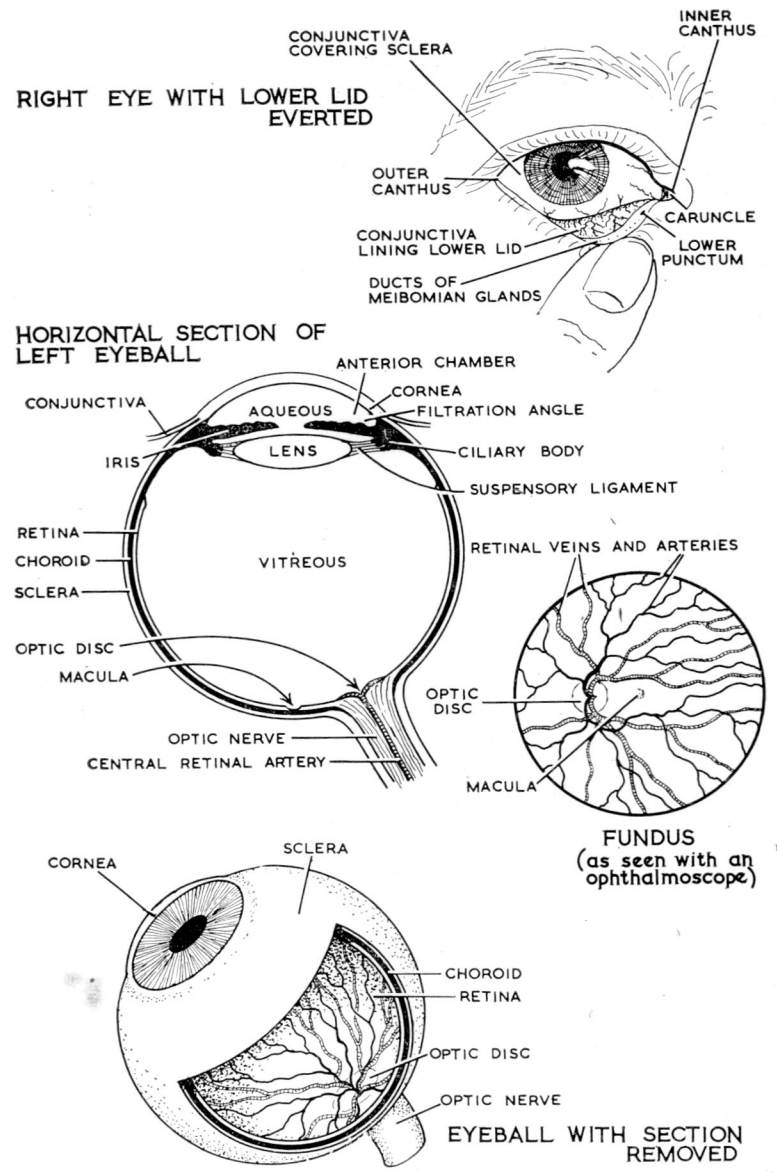

OPHTHALMIC NURSING

by

P. GARLAND

S.R.N., S.C.M., Ophthalmic Nursing Certificate of The Royal London Ophthalmic Hospital (Moorfield's Eye Hospital), Diploma in Nursing of the University of London, Sister Tutor's Certificate of the Royal College of Nursing. Formerly Sister in Charge of the Casualty and Outpatient Department, Sussex Eye Hospital, Brighton

FABER AND FABER
London

*First published in 1950
by Faber and Faber Limited
3 Queen Square London WC1
Second edition 1954
Third edition 1956
Fourth edition 1962
Fifth edition 1966
Revised impression 1968
Sixth edition 1975
Printed in Great Britain by
Latimer Trend & Company Ltd Plymouth
All rights reserved*

*ISBN 0 571 04872 2 (paper covers)
ISBN 0 571 04871 4 (hard-bound edition)*

CONDITIONS OF SALE

This book is sold subject to the condition that it shall not, by way of trade or otherwise, be lent, re-sold, hired out or otherwise circulated without the publisher's prior consent in any form of binding or cover other than that in which it is published and without a similar condition including this condition being imposed on the subsequent purchaser

© *Phyllis Garland 1975*

PREFACE TO FIRST EDITION

This book is intended for the general trained and student nurse rather than for those in ophthalmic hospitals.

The written word can never replace practical teaching, but a detailed description of nursing technique may be of value in a specialized branch of nursing in which experience is likely to be limited.

The aim has been to give full nursing details while as far as possible excluding anatomical and pathological descriptions; these are essential to intelligent nursing but are better dealt with by experts in appropriate textbooks. The detail which is included may appear superfluous but good nursing is dependent upon it and it is most frequently lacking when techniques are self-taught.

I wish to acknowledge my debt to all those from whom I learnt, and particularly to Miss D. E. Grand, formerly sister of the Ophthalmic Department of St. Thomas's Hospital. My grateful thanks are also due to Miss M. E. Gould, sister tutor, for her encouragement and criticism, and to Mr. P. G. Doyne, ophthalmic surgeon, for his help in the correction of medical errors in the text. The photographs are from various sources, and I should like to acknowledge the help given by St. Thomas's Hospital Photographic Department and by Mr. Dorset of Camera Talks. I am also grateful to Messrs. John Weiss for the numerous illustrations they have allowed me to use.

PREFACE TO FIFTH EDITION

In this edition there are a number of alterations and additions. I should like to thank all the staff of the Sussex Eye Hospital, Brighton, and in particular the surgeons, for their most helpful co-operation and for permission to include some pamphlets of advice which are used in the out-patient department. Some of the new photographs were taken by the photographer to this hospital group, and others are blocks kindly lent by various instrument makers and drug houses: C. W. Dixey & Son Ltd, Theodore Hamblin Ltd, Remploy Ltd, Smith & Nephew Pharmaceuticals Ltd, and John Weiss & Son Ltd.

As a result of my experience I am convinced that ophthalmic work is a most satisfying branch of nursing; it fulfils the need of many nurses to express themselves by manual dexterity, and provides opportunities for intelligent observation and for helping and advising patients in a practical way.

August 1966 P.G.

PREFACE TO SIXTH EDITION

In this edition there are further alterations and additions. Owing to my retirement from nursing, I have asked Mary Sharp for her help; she is the Nursing Officer in Charge of the Sussex Eye Hospital, Brighton, and Tutor to the Post-graduate students. We revised the nursing techniques in line with up-to-date surgery and the use of modern equipment, but we know that many small ophthalmic units work with less sophisticated methods and it is in these circumstances that a basic textbook is of particular value.

March 1974 P.G.

CONTENTS

Prefaces	*page* 5–7
1. Examination of eyes	19
2. Common eye treatments	32
3. Eye treatments *continued*	69
4. Investigations, Treatments and Minor Surgery	83
5. Bandages and Shades	107
6. Notes on Casualty and Outpatient Work	118
7. Nursing of In-patients	131
8. Cataract Nursing	136
9. Surgical Nursing *continued*	159
10. Notes on Ophthalmic Theatre work	192

Appendices

1. Eye Dressings and special Equipment	207
2. First Aid to the Eye	213
Glossary	217
Index	221

PLATES

I.	Ophthalmoscope	page 20
II.	Slit Lamp	21
III.	Slit Lamp in use	21
IV.	Lister Perimeter	28
V.	Bjerrum Screen	29
VI.	Edridge-Green Colour Perception Lantern	31
VII.	Book of Coloured Plates for Ishihara Test	31
VIII.	Light focused with a Convex Lens	33
IX.	Lids held open	33
X.	Eversion of upper lid (3 plates)	41
XI.	Eversion of upper lid using one hand only	43
XII.	'Minim' Packs of Eye Drops	45
XIII.	Instillation of Drops	57
XIV.	Application of Ointment with a glass rod	57
XV.	Application of Ointment from a tube	57
XVI.	Application of Ointment to a baby, using a rod	57
XVII.	Irrigation: the flow of lotion started on a cheek	64
XVIII.	Irrigation: the cheek dried before the undine is put down	64
XIX.	Irrigation for a baby	65
XX.	Steam Bathing an eye	71
XXI.	Hot Spoon Bathing	71
XXII.	Instructions for Steam Bathing an Eye	71
XXIII.	Epilation of Lashes	77
XXIV.	Painting the Conjunctiva with Silver Nitrate	78
XXV.	Expression of Lachrymal Sac	81

Plates

XXVI.	Syringing of Lachrymal Sac: insertion of the cannula	84
XXVII.	The taking of a Conjunctival Swab for Culture	86
XXVIII.	Scalpel Handle with Detachable Blades	92
XXIX.	Incision of Meibomian Cyst	92
XXX.	Corneal Lens and Haptic Lens	100
XXXI.	Boxes of Contact Lenses and their suction holders	101
XXXII.	Insertion of Haptic Contact Lenses	102
XXXIII.	The Removal of the Lens	102
XXXIV.	Placing the Corneal Contact Lens on the Eye (1)	103
XXXV.	Placing the Corneal Contact Lens on the Eye (2)	103
XXXVI.	Removal of the Corneal Contact Lens	104
XXXVII.	Single Eye Bandage I	109
XXXVIII.	Single Eye Bandage: alternative method I	109
XXXIX.	Single Eye Bandage II	109
XL.	Single Eye Bandage: alternative method II	109
XLI.	Single Eye Bandage III	109
XLII.	Double Eye Bandage	109
XLIII.	Knitted Eye Bandage	112
XLIV.	Moorfield's Double Eye Bandage	112
XLV.	Double Eye Elastoplast 'Gate' Dressing	113
XLVI.	An Adhesive Material used as an alternative to a bandage	113
XLVII.	Remploy Bathing Chair	133
XLVIII.	Occlusion applied to Spectacle Frame	180
XLIX.	Electric Hot-Air Sterilizer	193
L.	Sterilizer Box	194
LI.	Philps Giant Eye Magnet	196
LII.	Portable Magnet	197

LIST OF FIGURES

Diagrams of the Eye	*frontispiece*
Inspection Lamp	*page* 19
Test Type	23
'E' Test Type	24
Reading Test Type	26
Peripheral and Central Field Chart	27
Binocular loupe	34
Single corneal loupe	34
Anterior Chamber, normal and shallow	36
Hypopyon	36
Hyphaema, small and total	36
Pupil, fully dilated, pinpoint and irregular	37
Eversion of lower lid	41
Eversion of upper lid: eye closed, rod in position, lid everted	41
Rod under everted upper lid	42
Pipette	43
Drop Bottle with screw cap pipette	44
Plastic Drop Bottle	44
Drop Bottle Holders	46
Tissue Dispenser	47
Glass Eye Rod	56
Undine	60
Undine Stand	60
Fisher's Irrigation Tray	61
Mackintosh Cape	61
Patient lying with head at foot of bed for irrigation	62

List of Figures

Nurse standing behind chair and at side of bed	*page* 63
Covered Wooden Spoon	70
Electric Eye Warmer	73
Eye Warmer bandaged in position	73
Conjunctival Scissors	75
Epilation Forceps	76
Entropion of lower lid	80
Strapping for Entropion	80
Lids strapped closed	82
Punctum Dilator	83
Lachrymal Sac Cannula	83
Lachrymal Probe	84
Stitch Scissors (Long Iris)	88
Suture Forceps: Moorfield's pattern	88
Lang's Speculum	88
Lang's Lid Retractor	89
Corneal Foreign Body	89
Beer's Needle	90
Spud	90
Meibomian Clamp	93
Meibomian Curette	93
Schiotz tonometer with weights	97
Filter Paper inserted for Schirmer's Test	99
Knitted Bandage	111
Moorfield's Bandage	114
Pattern of Moorfield's Bandage	114
Many-tail Bandage	114
Cardboard Shade	115
Lint Flap	115
Celluloid Shield	115
Cartella Shield	115
Discission Needle, Saunder's	138
Keratome section	138
Keratome	138
Section for Extraction of Lens	138
Graefe Knife	139
Stages in Extraction of Lens	139

List of Figures

Cutting Lid Suture	*page* 147
Hyphaema	151
Iris Prolapse	152
Bowman's Needle	154
The Right and Wrong Way to put glasses down on a table	154
Corneal Graft Sutures	160
Drainage Angle	162
Visual examination of the iridic angle using the Goldmann gonioscopy lens	165
Small and large pupils	169
Conjunctival Flap	171
Retinal Detachment	174
Diagram showing how the 'string' is placed in the encircling string operation for retinal detachment	175
Right Convergent Squint	178
Spectacles for an Infant	180
Squint operation sutures	182
Artificial Eye	186
Removal of Artificial Eye	187
Lachrymal Apparatus	188
Knife Rack in tube	193
Mellinger's ring magnet	198
Haab's giant magnet	198
Hand magnet	198
Trial Drum	200
Trephine	200
Threading cotton through trephine	201
Sutures threaded on folded muslin	202
Folding Lint for Swabs	207
Sub-tarsal Foreign Body	214

PART I

I

EXAMINATION OF EYES

The examination of eyes usually takes place in a doctor's surgery or in a hospital casualty or out-patient department, but various types of eye-testing are undertaken in school clinics and in examination rooms where medical tests are carried out for entry to professions and armed services or for insurance purposes.

REQUISITES FOR EXAMINATION OF THE EYE BY A DOCTOR ARE:

Illumination can be provided by a pen torch but an inspection lamp run off the main electricity is very useful.

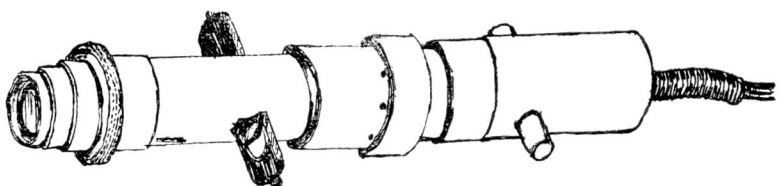

INSPECTION LAMP

Swabs or tissues and swabsticks will be necessary and cotton wool, as found in an eye-pad, to test corneal sensitivity.

Glass rods should be provided for eversion of eyelids.

Fluorescein paper strips or solution of fluorescein and drop bottles of normal saline to 'stain' the cornea (see page 54).

Examination of Eyes

The doctor usually has his own ophthalmoscope but otherwise one must be provided.

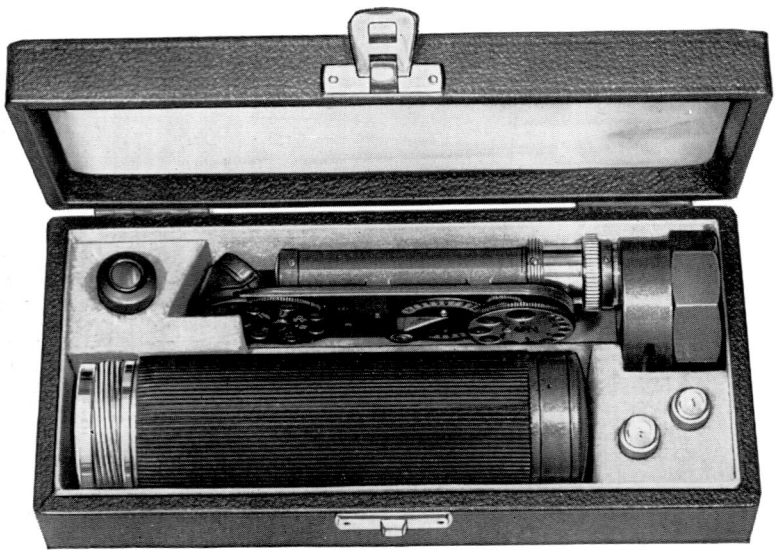

I. Ophthalmoscope

For *examination of the interior of the eyeball,* provision should be made to darken the surroundings if possible. Various instruments will be used, of which the ophthalmoscope (see plate I) is the most usual. Pantoscopes and indirect ophthalmoscopes allow more extensive examinations. Mydriatic drops such as homatropine, or a mixture of homatropine and cocaine, may be needed to dilate the pupil: these take twenty minutes to half an hour for a satisfactory effect and a miotic such as pilocarpine is usually instilled afterwards.

Slit-Lamp (see plates II and III)

A slit-lamp is a piece of equipment which combines a microscope with a lighting system which allows a source of light to be condensed into a narrow beam which is directed on to the front of

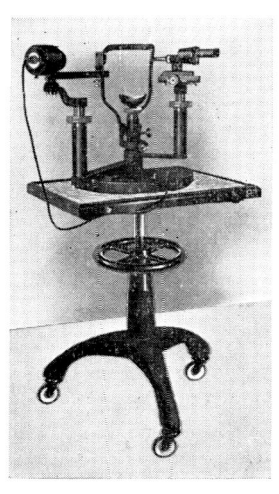 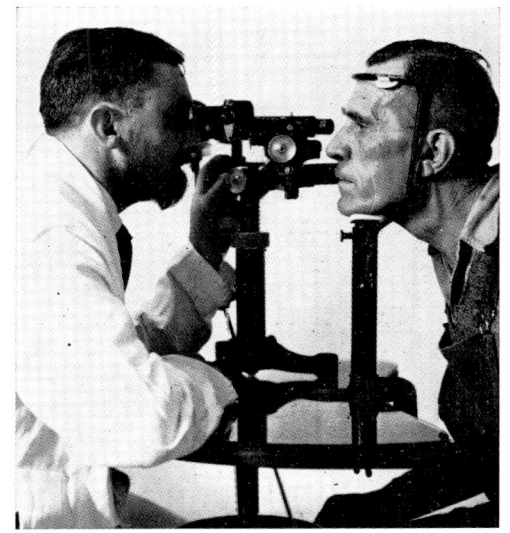

II. Slit lamp   III. The slit lamp in use. This examination would take place in a cubicle with dim lighting

the eye while the surrounding area is in dim light. The effect is as though a beam of sunlight is allowed into a dark room through a chink in the curtains and it makes it possible to see particles of dust which would be invisible in a room flooded with sunshine. With this concentrated illumination and the added magnification it is possible to examine the conjunctiva, cornea, anterior chamber, iris and lens. The slit-lamp is also used in combination with other equipment such as gonioscopes, pre-set lenses, contact lenses, and applanation tonometers. A slit-lamp should be in a dimly lit cubicle or corner of the examination room. It must be protected by a dust cover when not in use and the various screw adjustments should be kept lightly oiled. The microscope and lighting apparatus must be dusted and cleaned with particular care so as not to scratch the lenses or put the slit-lamp out of adjustment; soft tissues or a specially provided brush should be used. Slit-lamps vary from comparatively simple models to ones costing several hundred pounds.

Examination of Eyes

EXAMINATION OF CHILDREN

A doctor can often see a good deal of a small child's eye whilst he is talking to the mother with the child on her lap. It is always better for the nurse to be at hand but not to attempt to restrain a child unless asked to do so. With a co-operative child it is well worth remembering to warn him that drops will feel cold or that the first drop of cocaine will sting before making the eye numb. Children like being given a swab to hold so that they can mop their own eye afterwards. If it is necessary to hold him it is important that everything is in readiness so that the examination and treatment is as quick as possible. The mother should be where the child can see her; the assistant should spread a folded rug on the couch and then lie the child with his arms straight by his sides and wrap him securely in the rug. The assistant can sit on the couch by the child and steady his head, putting her hands each side of his cheeks with the thumbs under the chin. If help is needed to open an eye her index finger can control the lower lid without moving the hands. The confidence of children who are in-patients can usually be gained, but even then speed is a great point in successful treatment.

With a child in bed it is often difficult to prevent him rubbing a sore eye or disarranging the bandage: splinting of the arms is occasionally a necessary precaution: a straight splint is applied to the front of the arm, reaching above and below the elbow, thus preventing flexion.

TESTING VISUAL ACUITY

The tests for acuteness of central vision are those for distant vision, and near or reading vision. *Distant Vision* is tested at a distance of 20 feet (6 metres) since the rays of light from this distance are nearly parallel.

A Snellen's pattern test type consists of letters arranged on a chart, the size diminishing from above downwards. The top letter is of such a size that it can be read at 60 metres and then follow rows of letters which should be read at 36, 24, 18, 12, 9, 6, 5, and 4 metres respectively. The test type should be illuminated uniformly with standard lighting.

Examination of Eyes

The acuity of vision is expressed as a fraction, the numerator representing the number of metres the patient is from the chart, usually 6 metres, and the denominator the number indicating the distance at which the smallest letters read by the patient should be read by a normal eye. For instance, if the patient could only read 'CLOHNA' on the following chart his vision is recorded $V=6/9$. If he can read 'H' only it would be $V=6/60$. If he can read some letters in a line but not all it can be recorded as 'most' or 'part', for example, if he made two mistakes in the 6/5 line it would be 6/5 part. If the patient cannot see the largest letter from the 6 metre distance he can be walked slowly closer to the chart: If he sees the top letter at 3 metres $V=3/60$. If he cannot read the top letter at 1 metre he is tested with the examiner's hand held a foot away against a dark background and he is asked to count the number of fingers held up.

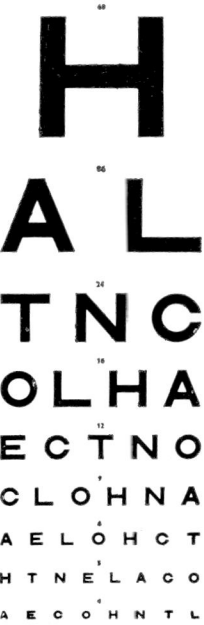

TEST TYPE

Examination of Eyes

If his answers are correct V=C.F. (count fingers at 1 foot). Should he not be able to count fingers the examiner moves his hand in front of the patient's eye; visual acuity would be recorded as V=H.M. (hand movements). These are good tests as no noise is made in putting up fingers or moving a hand. If he has less sight than this, the patient is tested with a torch in a dark or dimly lit room to see whether he can appreciate when illumination is on or off, and the vision is recorded as V=P.L. (perception of light), or V= No P.L. (no perception of light). To summarize the above, distant visual acuity ranges from 6/4 down to 6/60 and then from C.F., H.M., P.L., down to No P.L. which is total blindness.

If a length of 6 metres is not available for sight testing a test type of reversed letters may be used with a mirror. The chart is arranged just behind and above the patient's head and he reads the letters in a mirror placed at 3 metres in front of him.

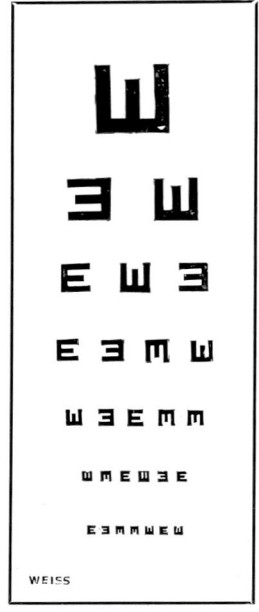

'E' TEST TYPE

Examination of Eyes

An illiterate chart can be used for a child, an illiterate person or one who does not know English letters. There are several different charts of which the 'E' is a well-known one. On the chart the 'E's' face in different directions and on some charts each 'E' can be turned by hand. The child holds a wooden 'E' and is asked to turn it the same way up as the one on the test chart to which the examiner is pointing.

Sheridan Gardner Test is another test which can be used for children. The test type has a single reversible letter on each line, e.g. O, H, V, T, and the child holds a card with these letters printed on it. He is asked to point to the letter on his card which corresponds to the letter on the test type. This test can be used for very young children as they do not have to name a letter.

In countries where the decimal system is in use the letters and distances are slightly different so that the readings are in multiples of ten and normal vision is 20/20.

Advice to a nurse who is testing visual acuity. As a rule the vision test is carried out by a doctor or an optician but a nurse may be responsible for doing it in certain circumstances as, for example, when she is assisting with routine medical examinations for employees or at a school clinic. In an eye hospital the nurses may do it on occasions such as when receiving casualty patients. The patient should be at 6 metres from the chart; each eye is tested separately, the other eye being covered by a card or cover held by the examiner. If the patient has glasses for constant use the vision of each eye should be tested first without glasses and then repeated with them, and both results should be recorded.

The following are difficulties which may arise during sight testing: the upper lid may be swollen so that the patient cannot open his eye; the nurse can usually raise it gently while the patient's head is tilted back to allow the letters to be read. If the eye is very painful or is watering profusely it may not be possible to get an accurate result and a note should be made accordingly. Occasionally a child or illiterate person will feel ashamed of not being able to read and will pretend they cannot see the letters, and, on the other hand, a man may be so keen to get a driving licence, or a boy to enter the Navy, that they learn all available charts by heart; if there is any doubt

Examination of Eyes

they can be asked to read the small letters backwards. When carrying out these tests the aim is to get the best possible result and encouragement and perseverance will often produce better results than are at first obtained.

The *Reading Test Type* is used for testing near vision.

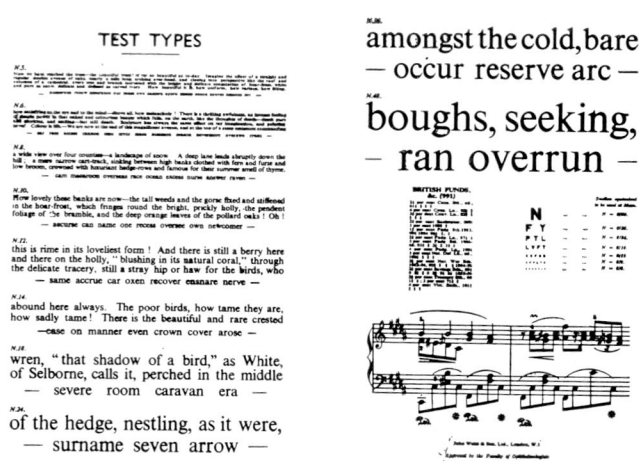

READING TEST TYPE

Near Vision is tested on test cards consisting of different sizes of ordinary printer's type and figures such as those in Stock Exchange columns. The patient should have a good light shining from behind his shoulder on to the card and the vision is recorded as the number of the smallest size type he can read. N5 is the smallest type on the standard test cards.

Fields of Vision

When the eye is fixed on some object there is a surrounding area of vision which is indistinct but of great value. The extent of this field of vision is limited by the surrounding structures of the eye such as the nose and orbit but when both eyes are being used the combined visual field is very wide. The physiological blind spot is due to

Examination of Eyes

the optic disc and is on the temporal side of the area of central vision: in a normal person who is looking with both eyes there is no blind spot in his field of vision because the right eye can see what would be on the blind spot of his left eye. The visual field is tested in two ways—firstly to find the extent or periphery of the field of each eye separately and secondly to examine the field for defects within the area of the field of vision. Neither of the tests is usually undertaken by nurses but an understanding of the importance of loss of field of vision, especially in glaucoma, adds to the interest a nurse takes in her part of the investigation and treatment.

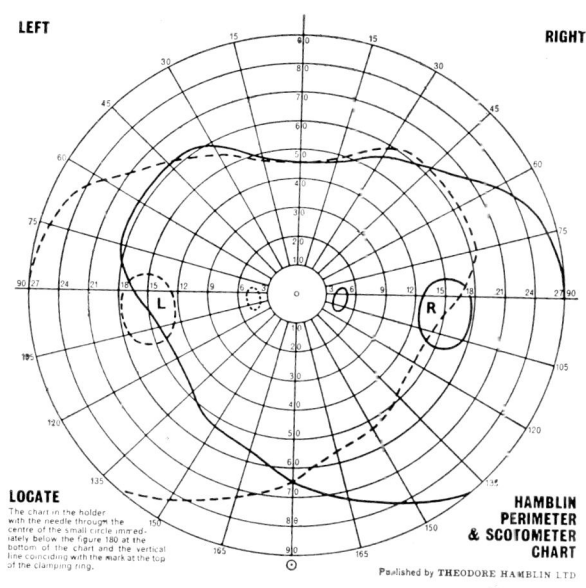

PERIPHERAL AND CENTRAL FIELD CHART

The field tests call for concentration on the part of the patient and it is usual to have the perimeter in a separate room or alcove off the main clinic room and to have provision for darkening the room so that the illumination on the perimeter holds the attention. Because a white uniform coat might distract the patient's attention a dark

Examination of Eyes

gown should be provided and a dark cotton sleeve for holding the target holder when doing central fields. There will need to be a cover or shield and pads for the eye not being examined, and coloured chalks or pens for drawing on the charts.

The *peripheral field* test is done with a perimeter (see plate IV). The instrument has an arc which will turn the full circle: the inner surface is black with a channel for a test object, which is usually white, to be moved slowly from the periphery in towards the centre. The patient sits with his head kept in the correct position by having his chin in the chin rest. He is asked to look at the central white fixation spot and indicate when he can see the test object being

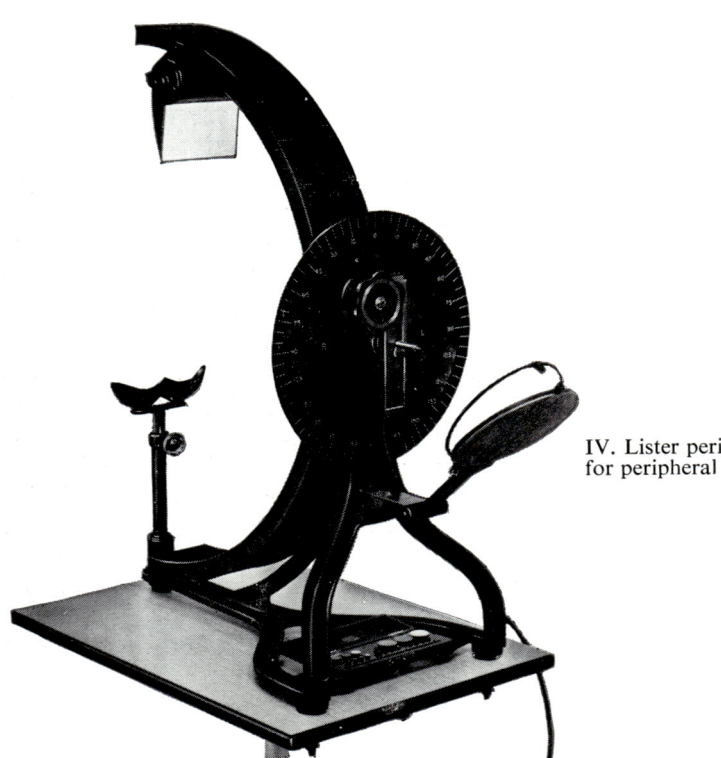

IV. Lister perimeter for peripheral fields

Examination of Eyes

brought in from the periphery. The arc is moved round at intervals of five degrees of the circle and the instrument has a device for recording the position of the test object when it is seen by the patient. The recording consists of a circle of pricked holes on a chart and these marks are then connected to give the outline of the patient's field of vision for comparison with the normal one. The second eye is covered while one is tested.

The Goldmann Perimeter is also used for peripheral field tests. This is a complicated piece of equipment and the person carrying out the test must be specially trained.

The Bjerrum Screen (see plate V) is used for examining the central part of the field of vision. The screen consists of a large piece of

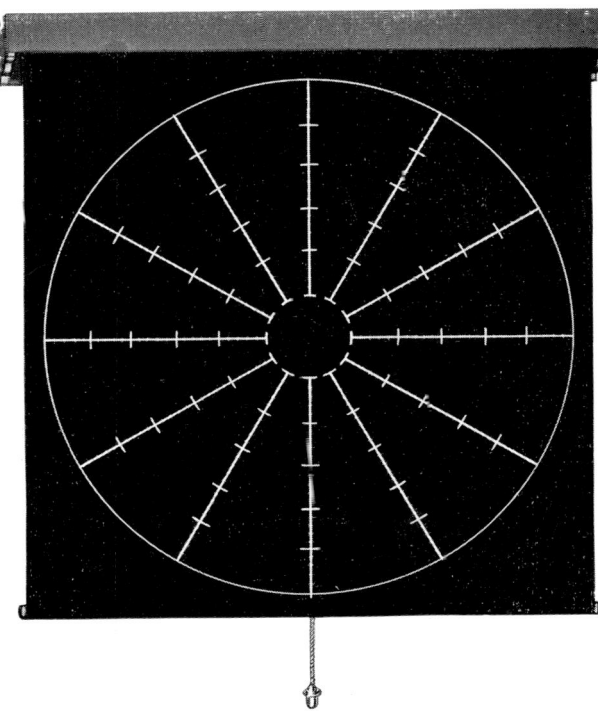

V. Bjerrum screen 2 metres square for central fields

Examination of Eyes

black material 2 metres square with a white spot in the centre and concentric rings of black stitching at certain intervals and also radiating lines of stitching. These markings are not visible to the patient but they are reproduced on the special chart on which the doctor plots out the normal blind spot and any abnormalities. The examination is carried out in a darkened room with special illumination for the screen. The patient sits 2 metres from it and the test is done with white or coloured test objects which are very small discs or balls fixed on to the end of a long black stick. The object is moved over the screen and the patient asked to keep looking at the centre fixed spot and say when the test object disappears from his field of vision. Each eye is tested separately. It is a subjective test and it is often by no means easy to evaluate the accuracy of the result.

A visual fields analyser can be used for examining the central field of vision. The screen has small holes in it which can be made to light up in various sequences. The patient tells the operator how many lights he sees in each sequence and the result is recorded on a special chart.

For the purpose of watching the control of glaucoma the value of the field tests is largely in the comparison of tests done at successive intervals and it is most important that the charts should have the patient's name and medical number and the date clearly on each chart so that they can be traced if they get separated from the medical notes; the entry on each chart will also include indication of the size and colour of the target used.

In circumstances where a nurse is required to do field of vision tests special instruction will be given, and if any abnormality is found which was not present on a previous test the doctor should be consulted as to whether he wishes to check the findings.

Colour Vision

The ability to recognize colours may be essential for some occupations and particularly for those which involve the use of colour signals such as road traffic lights and navigational signals. There are various tests for colour vision some of which make use of a lantern (see plate VI) in which an aperture provides for different colours and combinations of colours to be shown with variations in intensity

Examination of Eyes

of lighting. The test in general use is the Ishihara one; this is a book of coloured plates (see plate VII) in which various numbers are shown in different colours against a background of confusion dots. There is an explanatory table which shows the charts normal people can see whereas those who are colour blind read a different number.

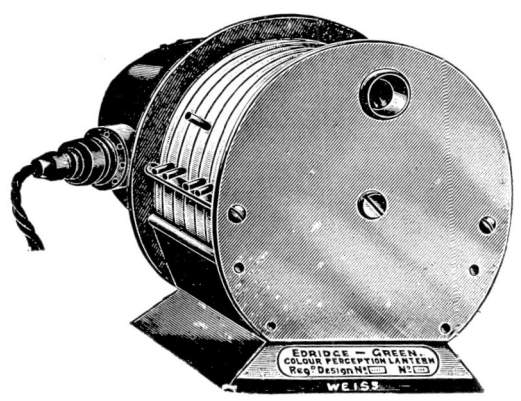

VI. Edridge-Green colour perception lantern

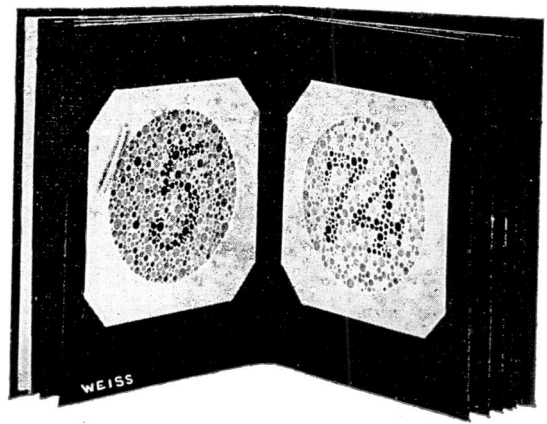

VII. Book of coloured plates for Ishihara test

2

COMMON EYE TREATMENTS

The handling of eyes is of the greatest importance. A gentle and yet firm touch is required; rough and jerky movements are frightening, but indecisive and ineffectual ones are the commoner failing and to the patient they are a source of irritation and loss of confidence.

Training in correct technique is necessary, but over and above this a certain amount of practice is essential before a nurse can become skilful.

A good light is essential for the observation of as small a structure as the eye. Daylight is excellent and for preference the patient should be arranged facing a window. If this is not possible for a bed patient, additional lighting will usually be necessary, a narrow beam from a bright light is ideal. A pen torch is satisfactory but a bell lamp or a large torch with a half-used battery are too diffuse unless the beam is concentrated with a convex lens (see plate VIII). Special electric ophthalmic lamps are ideal if the wiring allows them to be plugged in over each bed (see inspection lamp on page 19).

Magnification can be obtained with corneal loupes, but some practice is required if they are to be used with advantage (see p. 34).

TO HOLD AN EYE OPEN

No patient can open his eye satisfactorily in a bright light and the lid must be held for him. Any pressure on the eyeball is uncomfortable and if the eye is inflamed it will be very painful; therefore the lids must be held against the bony orbital ridge where the patient will not mind firm pressure (see plate IX).

VIII. Light focused with a convex lens

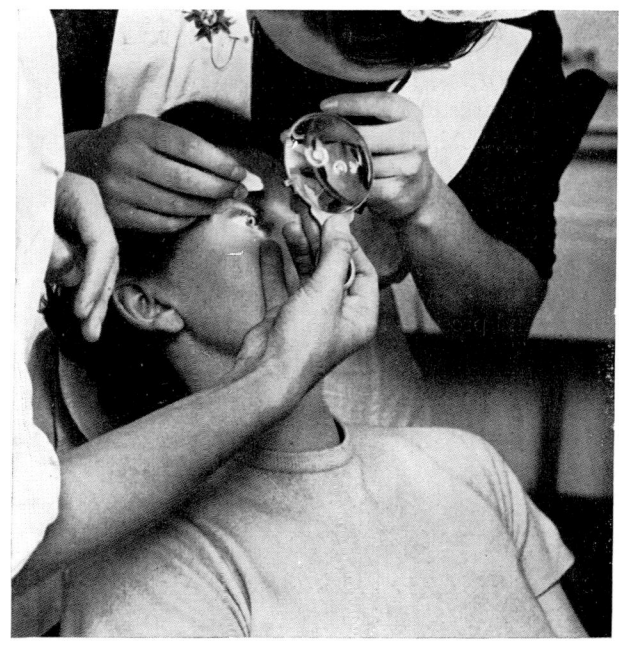

IX. Lids held open. The loose skin of the lids is being pressed against the upper and lower orbital ridge to avoid any pressure on the eyeball

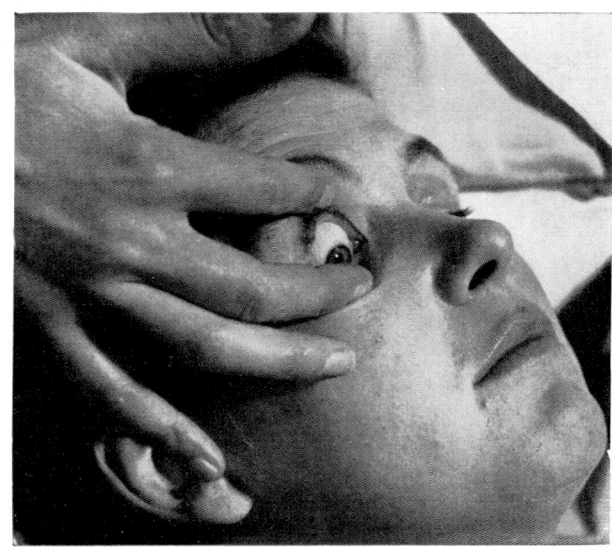

Common Eye Treatments

To hold the lower lid the patient is asked to look up, the tip of the finger is placed just below the lashes in the centre of the lid, and the loose skin is drawn gently down and then pressed firmly against the bone. With *the upper lid* it is more difficult to prevent pressure on the eye. The patient looks down, the finger is put as close to the lashes as possible and the loose skin of the lid is drawn upwards and again held firmly against bone. There is a great difference between this method and the practice of placing a finger flat on the upper lid and pressing back into the orbit.

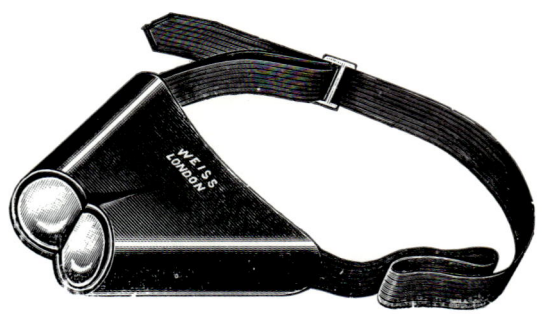

BINOCULAR LOUPE

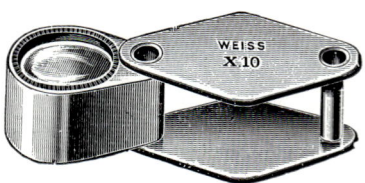

SINGLE CORNEAL LOUPE

It can be very difficult to get a grip on lids which are greasy from the application of ointment.

When opening *a baby's lids* great care must be taken that the cornea is not scratched by a finger-nail. If conjunctivitis is present the scratch is particularly likely to become infected with the most serious consequences to the baby's sight. For this reason the nurse's

Common Eye Treatments

finger-nails must be kept short and the tip of the finger be just behind the edge of the lid.

HOLDING THE LIGHT

If artificial light is used the lamp should be held about four inches from the face, the light being first brought on to the cheek and then up to the eye, the patient having been warned. The light must not be kept on the eye for a moment longer than while it is being used, as it is very tiring for the patient.

METHOD OF INSPECTION OF AN EYE

For accurate observation the nurse should practise looking at an eye methodically so that nothing is missed on the single occasion.

The following points should first be noted:

Whether the eye has been comfortable. If painful, whether the pain is increasing or decreasing and the character of the pain, e.g. 'aching pain', 'shooting pain', 'pain round the eye', etc. In reference to the latter point the patient should be asked to describe it himself rather than have it suggested to him.

OBSERVATIONS TO BE MADE

1. If the eye is covered *the pad* may be wet, or discharge may be present; the type of discharge should be noted.

2. *The lids* may be red or swollen or tender.

3. *The lashes* may be crusted.

4. On opening the eye *the conjunctiva* is normally white but it may be injected (red) or chemosed. Chemosis is oedema of the conjunctiva which is so loosely attached to the underlying sclera that the fluid causes the conjunctiva to swell out with a ballooned appearance.

5. *The Cornea* is normally transparent but it may be hazy or opaque rendering it impossible to see the iris and pupil.

6. *The Anterior Chamber* (A.C.) is the space between the cornea in front and the iris behind and is filled with the fluid aqueous; if too little aqueous is present the iris appears to be pressed up against the cornea and it is described as a 'shallow anterior chamber' (an infant's eye has normally a very shallow anterior chamber). The aqueous may be cloudy, in which case the iris cannot be seen clearly.

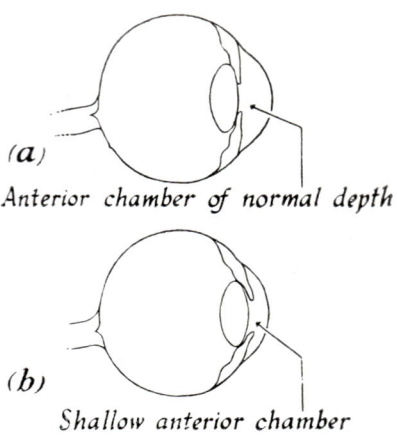

(a) Anterior chamber of normal depth

(b) Shallow anterior chamber

Foreign material may be present in the anterior chamber; this may be blood (hyphaema), or pus (hypopyon). Pus is seldom present in large quantity, but blood may vary from a streak at the bottom of the A.C. to a 'total hyphaema' in which the A.C. is filled with blood.

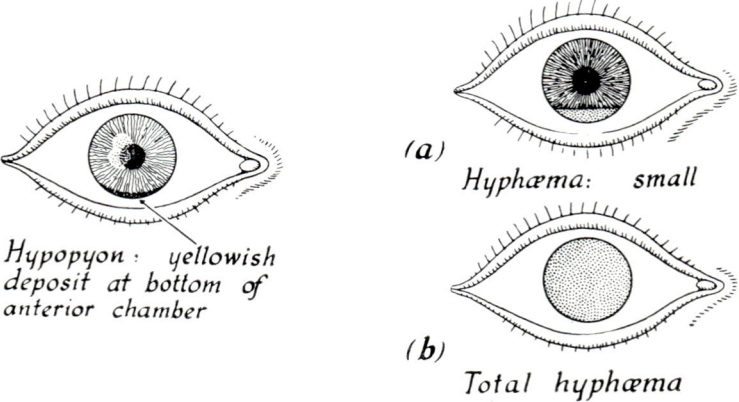

Hypopyon: yellowish deposit at bottom of anterior chamber

(a) Hyphæma: small

(b) Total hyphæma

7. *The Iris.* The normal colour should be that of the healthy eye. It may be dull and 'muddy'.

The iris should react by the pupil contracting briskly to a bright

Common Eye Treatments

light; it may be sluggish or fail to contract. If miotic or mydriatic drops are being used it is obviously impossible to observe the reaction to light.

8. *The Pupil*. The degree of dilatation and the shape of the pupil must be noted.

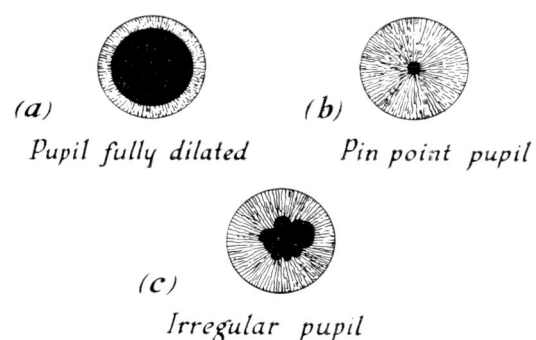

(a) Pupil fully dilated *(b) Pin point pupil*

(c) Irregular pupil

9. *Photophobia* (fear of light) or excessive *lachrymation* (watering) should be noted.

10. *The vision of the eye* is not usually tested when inspecting it, but any comment by the patient regarding improvement or deterioration may be significant.

A nurse should practise looking at every eye in this way so that she can report any abnormality on either point, improvement or deterioration, and also the effect of treatment which is given, e.g. if the pupil is dilated after the use of atropine drops.

MODIFIED METHODS OF ASEPTIC TECHNIQUE

The nurse's hands must be dry, not only because of the bacteriological danger of wet hands, but also on account of the discomfort to the patient.

For out-patient work it is considered adequate if the hands are washed thoroughly between treatments and are dried in a warm air drier or on disposable towels or freshly laundered towels.

For ward patients more rigid care is always required owing to the fact that they are more seriously ill and consequently have a lower

Common Eye Treatments

resistance to infection: also a hospital ward is a particularly rich source of bacteriological infection. The 'no-touch' technique is very difficult to carry out in eye work as the eyelids must be held during treatments, and it does not seem possible to handle them properly with forceps. During nearly all treatments a swab is held on the lower lid to prevent tears running down the cheek and to catch an overflow of drops, and this swab must be touched by the fingers. At the present time most eye hospitals and departments allow the nurse to touch the swabs and eyelids, but in the cases of acute infection and in the early dressings after intraocular operations, the hands are washed particularly thoroughly and dried on a sterilized towel. There is the possibility of using sterilized gloves, but it is not widely practised. It seems more sensible to concentrate on a good dressing technique, for example, nurses are taught never to use the same side of a swab a second time and not to touch that part of the eye pad which is to come in contact with the lids.

This technique seems contradictory to general surgical principles and so is difficult for the student nurse, but it must be remembered that the eyeball is covered by the lids and the tears contain lysozyme which has some bactericidal action.

Dressings. It is ideal if individual packets of sterilized dressings are used for each patient but if these are not available the dressings may be autoclaved in small drums or boxes.

Instruments. Again it is ideal to have them dry sterilized in individual packs (see page 209) but if this is not possible they should be boiled for three minutes, or for the time required by the individual hospital rules, both before and after use; this does not apply to knives, the blades of which are ruined by even the most careful boiling; they should be placed in a special rack and immersed in disinfectant solution for the required time. Sharp instruments can be sterilized in individual packs in hot-air ovens. (See page 199 for care of theatre instruments.)

SWABBING EYES

Even if there is no discharge from an eye, if it is bandaged, an eye pad often makes the skin irritable and the lids require to be swabbed once a day or oftener. The lotion ordered may be normal saline, but

Common Eye Treatments

boiled water can be used; sodium bicarbonate solution will help to soften and remove crusted discharge.

Swabs may be of white lint, or cotton wool balls, or special gauze swabs which contain a very thin layer of wool. The swab should be folded to form a firm pad and only the tip be dipped in the lotion. It should be squeezed so that it is damp and not dripping, care being taken to avoid touching the tip with the fingers.

The lower lid usually needs the most attention and, with the patient looking up, it is swabbed from the nasal corner outwards; in this direction because of the danger of swabbing discharge into the lachrymal punctum or in a baby it would be easy to wipe discharge over the bridge of the nose into the other eye. The amount of pressure required is difficult to describe, but it must be gentle and yet firm. The edge of the swab must not be above the lid margin for fear of touching the sensitive cornea.

When the lashes of the *upper lid* are crusted they can be swabbed more effectively if the lid margin is slightly everted; with the patient looking down a light brushing action with the damp swab will remove the discharge. Lids crusted as the result of *blepharitis* need more thorough treatment; they are best dealt with by firm rubbing with a prepared swab stick moistened with lotion; these lids require patient and thorough care to remove all crusts before the prescribed treatment can be effectively applied. As the patients are often small children, mothers find it a most difficult procedure at home and treatment as an in-patient for a few days will often work wonders.

Ointment which has previously been applied to the skin of the lids is most easily removed with paraffin or olive oil.

EVERSION OF EYELIDS (see plate X)

It is often necessary to expose the conjunctival surface of the eyelids, e.g. for the removal of foreign bodies or to treat the conjunctiva.

Eversion of the Lower Lid. This is very easy to evert. The lid is drawn down and the patient is asked to look up: with a little manipulation all the folds of the conjunctiva can be brought into view.

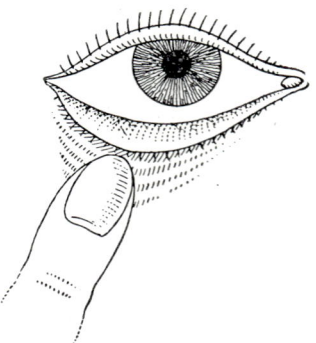

EVERSION OF LOWER LID

Eversion of the Upper Lid. The eversion of the upper lid needs a little practice after the method has been learnt, but it is essential for a nurse to acquire the ability. It is advisable to practise on a healthy eye as the patient with the foreign body cannot help screwing up his eye and making it a little more difficult. As in other eye treatments, the discomfort comes from pressure on the eyeball; this is minimized if the lid is drawn down and away from the eye so that pressure with the glass rod, to depress the upper border of the tarsal plate, is made

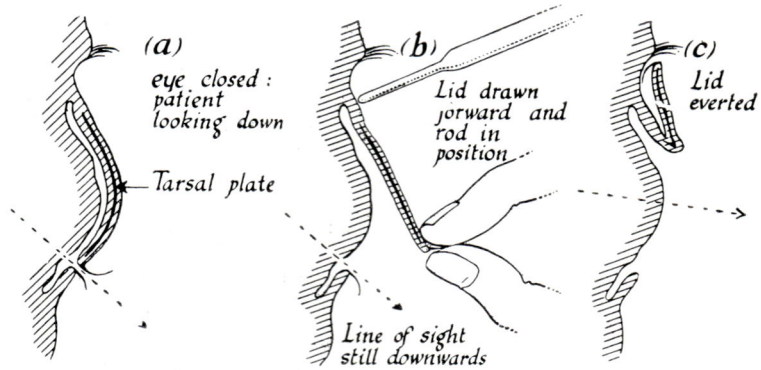

EVERSION OF UPPER LID: (*a*) EYE CLOSED, (*b*) ROD IN POSITION, (*c*) LID EVERTED

X. Eversion of upper eyelid

i) The lashes are held between the first finger and thumb, to draw the lid down and away from the eyeball, directing the patient to look down

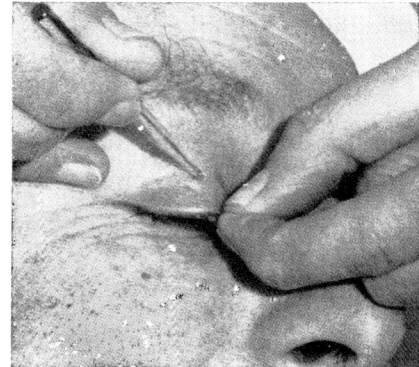

ii) With a glass rod depressing the lid at the upper margin of the tarsal plate the eyelid is turned over, using the tip of the rod as a fulcrum

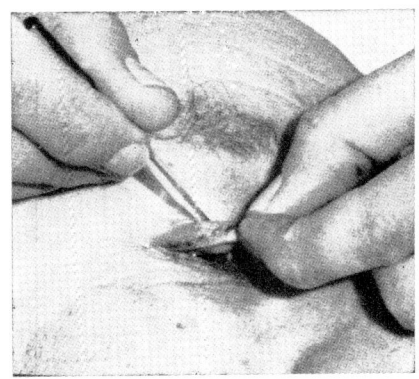

iii) The lid is kept everted by pressing the lashes or lid margin against the skin of the lid, and asking the patient to keep looking down

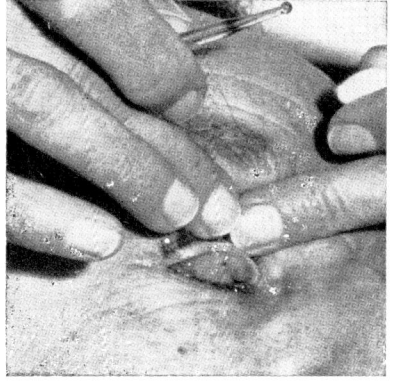

Common Eye Treatments

on to the space between the lid and the eye. The lashes of the upper lid are held between the first finger and thumb to draw the lid down. The patient *must look down to his toes* or the tarsal plate will not be in view. When the lid is everted, the retrotarsal space is still hidden.

Eversion of lid and examination of retrotarsal fold

When the upper lid is everted there is still a space in the upper fornix which is not seen and it may be necessary to inspect it. After putting in a few local anaesthetic drops, the retrotarsal fold can be exposed by slipping a glass rod under the edge and then lifting it as the rod is moved along.

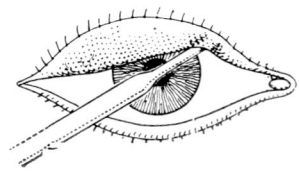

ROD UNDER EVERTED UPPER LID

Eversion of the upper lid using one hand (see plate XI)

This method requires practice, and should not be used on a patient until the knack has been acquired, as it is a little more uncomfortable for the patient, even when skilfully done. It is of great advantage when irrigation of the everted lid is necessary and it is the only method possible if the eyelashes have been cut or if they are very scanty. Lids which are slightly swollen by inflammation turn over much more easily, and a baby's lid will evert readily.

The method is shown and described on plate XI.

THE INSTILLATION OF EYE DROPS

Eye drops are used for treatment of the external structures of the eye but they are also absorbed through the cornea to affect the inside of the eyeball, e.g. atropine drops cause the pupil to dilate.

Drop Bottles

There is a variety of different patterns of droppers and drop bottles.

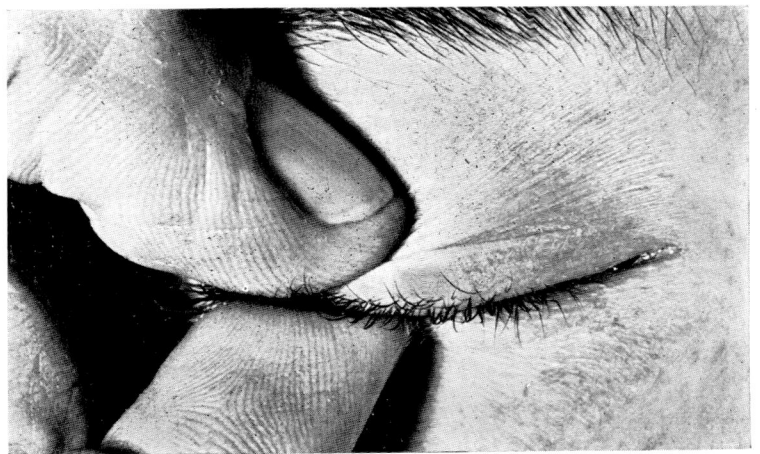

XI. Eversion of the upper lid

This is a description of the method using one hand only: standing behind or to the side of the patient who is instructed to look down, the first finger is placed at the outer end of the lower lid and draws the lid slightly away from the outer side of the orbit. At the same time the thumb presses on the margin of the upper lid to draw it also outwards and allow the lower lid to be rolled under it. When the tarsal plate of the upper lid can be felt between the finger and thumb the lid is everted with a rotary movement

PIPETTE

Pipettes. These are easy to use, but they should be dry sterilized or boiled between each treatment as it is difficult to keep them sterile between use. Disposable pipettes are available but they are expensive at present. The shorter the pipette the more control there is over the direction of the drop.

BOTTLE WITH PIPETTE INCORPORATED IN THE STOPPER

Advantages. There is complete control of the flow of the drops by pressure on the pipette.

Disadvantages. The solution will be contaminated if the pipette has touched either the patient's lashes or the outside of the bottle

Common Eye Treatments

when being replaced. For the use of an individual patient or in special hospitals the risk is probably negligible, but in inexperienced hands this is a definite consideration. The rubber caps need frequent replacement.

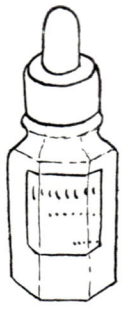

DROP BOTTLE WITH
SCREW CAP PIPETTE

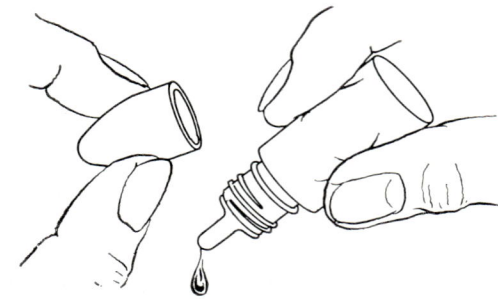

PLASTIC DROP BOTTLE

PLASTIC BOTTLES

The drop bottle above right is a plastic one.

The advantage is that no pipette is required as the soft plastic material allows the bottle to be squeezed to expel a drop. They are made by the individual drug houses supplying the solutions and are, therefore, more expensive and the bottle is labelled with the trade name of the solution. Oily drops are convenient to use from this type of bottle or from individual packs. (See plate XII.)

Research is being undertaken to design better drop bottles; the special requirements are, that the bottles can be adequately sterilized, that the flow of drops can be properly controlled and that the contents of the bottle cannot be easily contaminated. It sometimes proves best for hospital work that a freshly sterilized pipette be taken for each patient and be discarded immediately; the problem includes the designing of a suitable cover or stopper for the bottle between use, and of a convenient container from which sterile pipettes can be taken.

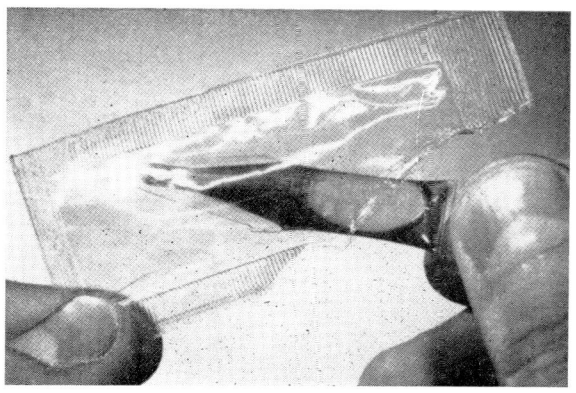

XII. *'Minim' Packs of Eye Drops*
These packs contain sufficient solution for one application, and therefore have the advantage that there is no risk of contamination of a drop bottle. They would be most useful if the quantity required was not large, but would prove an expensive way of supplying an eye hospital

INSTILLATION OF DROPS

The aim is to put the required number of drops inside the eyelids with the minimum of discomfort to the patient and without letting any fall on the skin of the cheek.

The problem when using drop bottles is that two hands are needed to hold the bottle steady and pick up the pipette; if the bottle can be held securely, one hand only is necessary. It is also likely that bottles fall over and spill when in use if the cap holding the pipette is not screwed on between treatments.

The stand (see p. 46) should preferably be weighted and have felt on the bottom to prevent movement. Care must be taken that the spring clips are not in a position to cover the label on the bottle.

The number of drops to be instilled depends on the type of solution. As a general rule, one drop is sufficient if it falls in properly; no harm can be done by putting in several drops and if there is the least doubt if the first one went in, more should be instilled. Nurses need reassuring on the point that this is not exceeding the dose as it would

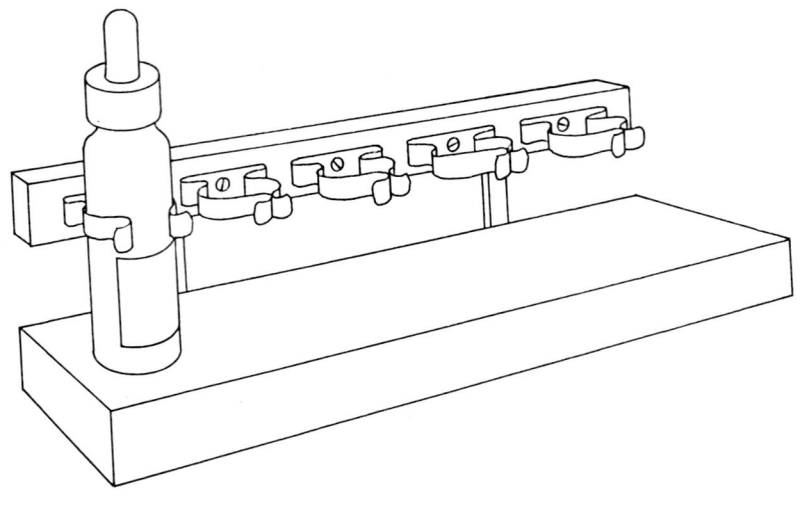

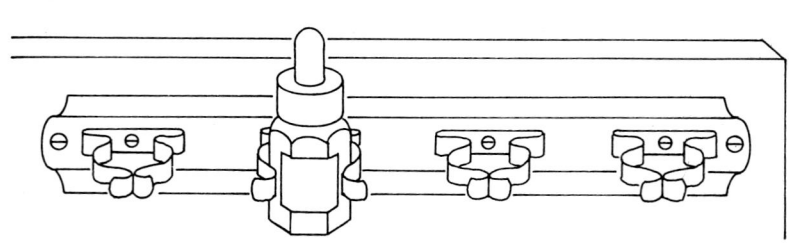

DROP BOTTLE HOLDERS

The metal strip, on which the spring clips are screwed, can be attached to the front of a stationery rack on a desk, or to any convenient place.

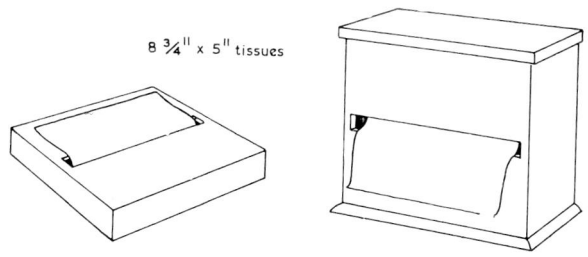

TISSUE DISPENSER

Small tissues are ideal for use as a swab when putting in drops. Dispensers for the boxes can be fixed to a desk or wall for clinic use.

be in the case of a drug given by other routes. There are some exceptions to this rule. They are as follows:

Oily Solutions, e.g. Paroleine, are used for lubrication of the eye and therefore several drops should be put in at each application.

Anaesthetic drops, e.g. cocaine, act according to the quantity instilled, and it is usual to put in two or three at a time, this being continued at a few minute intervals until they are not felt as they drop on the eye. Some eyes will need much more cocaine than others. While being cocainized, the eye must be kept shut as it has the effect of drying the cornea and making it hazy.

The drops should be put into the outer side of the lower fornix. The conjunctiva is less sensitive than the cornea and the outer side is preferable as the punctum of the tear apparatus is situated at the nasal end.

To treat conditions of the lachrymal passages, it is hoped that the drop will pass into the punctum and therefore the drop should fall as near to it as possible.

For corneal conditions, lubricating drops should fall on to the cornea; the patient will not object in this case as oily drops do not feel cold like watery ones.

For local anaesthesia, the first drops should be put into the lower fornix and the subsequent ones directly onto the eyeball.

Common Eye Treatments

The position of the dropper should be as close to the eye as possible without touching the lids—about an inch away. If drops fall from a height they are more uncomfortable and their destination is less easily controlled; it is equally important that the dropper must not be contaminated or the eyeball touched. In the instance of a child who might move, it is safer to hold the dropper a little farther away.

The position of the patient's head is of primary importance. It must be resting back with the chin up. This is possible in an ordinary chair, the patient being asked to put his head back, but if difficulty is experienced the head must be supported by a chair with a head rest or by the patient lying down. If the patient is in bed, the pillows must be arranged so that his head rests comfortably.

In a private house an armchair is often very suitable.

A small child should be lying down and securely held.

General Instructions

The label on the bottle should be checked with the prescription.

The drops ought to be ordered for the right or left eye and the nurse should query it if this is not stated and there is the least doubt.

The bottle or dropper should be tested to ascertain how easily the drop will fall.

The patient's head must be in the correct position.

A folded swab should be placed on the lower lid right up to the lash margin.

At the moment when the drop is falling, the patient should be asked to look up and the lower lid be drawn down so that the drop falls to the outer side of the lower fornix (see plate XIII, p. 57).

The swab must be kept on the lower lid until the patient has closed his eye and the excess of tears has been absorbed by the swab.

Warnings

Eye drops must not be warmed before use. It is sometimes suggested that they would be less uncomfortable if warm but many of them are chemically unstable when heated, with the result that they may become ineffective and an irritant to the eye.

The upper lid should not be touched if the patient is able to open the eye himself. If it is necessary to raise it for him, as in the case of

Common Eye Treatments

an unconscious or deaf patient, or a small child, the swab should be held on the lower lid with the second finger while the first is used to lift the upper lid at the moment when the drop falls.

The patient must not be asked to look up or the lower lid be drawn down until the drop is ready to fall; this may sound unnecessary advice but, with the pneumatic type of bottle, it is a common mistake to have the patient looking up for quite a long time, and it will be more of a shock when the drop eventually comes, or else he will have become tired and shut the eye.

Drops should not be allowed to fall on the skin; it is uncomfortable and with some drops, e.g. atropine, it may encourage a skin irritation which makes it impossible to continue with the drops.

It cannot be stressed too often that the drop will never fall in if the head is too erect.

Witnessing of Drops

It is a wise precaution in a general hospital, to witness miotic drops, e.g. eserine and pilocarpine. These drugs cannot do serious harm, but they are ordered for a glaucomatous eye which might be irreparably damaged by a mydriatic given in error. In this connection it must be mentioned that special care should be taken if the second eye is being treated with a mydriatic. Atropine is a particularly powerful drug and would be effective if the least quantity got in from a contaminated finger or swab, or from the dropper being held in such a way that a drop could fall into the wrong eye. For this reason it may be wise, in certain circumstances, to witness atropine. Should a mistake occur, an immediate report to the surgeon will allow counter measures to be taken whereas delay might be fatal to the patient's sight. Some pharmacists use labels of a distinguishing colour for mydriatic and miotic drops.

NOTES ON EYE DROPS IN COMMON USE

Drops for the eye are termed *guttae*.

The drops can be divided into groups according to their action on the eye.

Common Eye Treatments

Mydriatic Drops

Mydriatics dilate the pupil; they are usually also cycloplegics—by paralysis of the ciliary muscle, they prevent the lens being able to accommodate for near vision. Their chief uses are:

(*a*) In the prevention and treatment of diseases of the uveal tract, e.g. iritis, choroiditis and cyclitis.

(*b*) For ophthalmoscopic examination of the fundus.

(*c*) For refraction of the eye.

Atropine sulphate $\frac{1}{2}$–2 per cent is the most powerful mydriatic and frequently used.

It takes a few hours for the maximum effect to be obtained. In a healthy eye there is some degree of dilatation for at least a week; for this reason it is uneconomical for use after minor injuries, as close work is interfered with while the eye is under the effect of the drug.

No miotic drop will counteract atropine, and therefore it is not used for examination of the fundus except in children: in elderly patients continued dilatation might precipitate an attack of glaucoma.

Atropine Irritation. This is sometimes caused and has the appearance of a local inflammation around the eye, the skin becoming red and swollen with a serous exudation resembling eczema. It is a very troublesome condition as the mydriatic is often essential to the eye. It is usually treated with steroid preparations and if cream or ointment are used they should be applied before the drops, as they form a protective covering to the skin. If the irritation persists the mydriatic is changed. If available in the form of lamellae, the drug will be less likely to cause irritation.

Patients having atropine regularly, occasionally complain of a dry throat; the tendency is reduced by the instillation of the drop to the outer side of the lower fornix thus lessening the chance of its passing down the lachrymal passages to the throat.

Atropine is sometimes held to be responsible for mental confusion in the aged.

Phenylephrine, 10 per cent is less powerful than atropine but it dilates the pupil fully and can be neutralized by miotic drops such as pilocarpine or eserine.

Homatropine hydrobromide, $\frac{1}{2}$–2 per cent, is very commonly used

Common Eye Treatments

for rapid dilatation of the pupil for examination purposes. It is frequently combined with cocaine, 1 per cent: its effect can be neutralized with miotic drops.

Mydrilate 1 *per cent* (*cyclopentolate*) will dilate a pupil in about fifteen minutes and its effect is easily reversed by eserine, and it is therefore of value for examination of the fundus. Cycloplegia is produced in adults in fifteen minutes and in children in forty minutes, and it is a useful alternative to other drugs for refraction.

There are a number of other mydriatic drops including solutions of a mixture of various mydriatics. Hyoscine, and E3 or Lachesine, are sometimes tried if atropine irritation occurs.

Miotic Drops

These contain drugs which contract the pupil.

They are used in the treatment of glaucoma and to counteract the effect of homatropine. Sometimes they are ordered after cataract operation.

Eserine sulphate (Physostigmine), $\frac{1}{8}$–1 per cent, decomposes in light to a reddish colour and is then ineffective and irritant: for this reason it is often dispensed in dark glass bottles and when not in use it should be kept in a cupboard.

In cases of acute glaucoma, eserine may be ordered 'intensively'; then it is often combined with local heat and may be put in at five minute intervals for half an hour. The strongest solution is 1 per cent in castor oil.

The regular use of eserine may irritate the eye, causing some conjunctivitis and, more rarely, nausea and general discomfort. Patients complain of a 'dragging' feeling when it is used after a mydriatic.

Pilocarpine nitrate, $\frac{1}{4}$–4 per cent, is less powerful than eserine, but it is not so irritant and is often used regularly in mild glaucoma.

Phospholine iodide is a miotic drop sometimes used in open-angle glaucoma, but it has been known to produce side-effects.

Local Anaesthetic Drops

These drops anaesthetize the eye and the inner surface of the lids

A congested eye requires very much more local anaesthetic and it may not be possible to render it completely insensitive with drops.

Common Eye Treatments

The nurse should warn the surgeon if she has not been able to anaesthetize the eye properly.

The quantity of local anaesthetic drops required varies with different patients and for different procedures. For the removal of a superficial foreign body, one drop may be effective in two minutes. For an operation it is usually ordered half an hour beforehand: two or three drops should be put in at intervals of a few minutes until the patient cannot feel them going in, and then at five-minute intervals until operation, the eyes being kept closed between instillations. Just before the surgeon commences one drop is put into the other eye to help the patient to keep it open.

Local anaesthetic drops before operation must always be ordered specifically to the right or left eye as there may well be doubt as to which one the surgeon intends to operate upon, for example, in squint or cataract cases.

There is a school of thought which considers that an eye which has been rendered insensitive must be covered for an hour or two, as the patient will blink less frequently to moisten the eyeball, and will not feel if a foreign body should enter it.

Cocaine hydrochloride, 2–4 per cent, is the most commonly used and the most powerful: 4 per cent is the usual strength. It must be specially ordered as a drug coming under the Misuse of Drugs Act.

In addition to its anaesthetic action it causes dilatation of the pupil and for this reason is often combined with homatropine. Cocaine has a desiccating action on corneal epithelium causing superficial opacity and therefore it is especially important that the eye be kept closed between instillations. The patient should be warned that the first drops will sting slightly before having a numbing effect: sometimes a 2 per cent solution is used to start with, but it is doubtful if it makes an appreciable difference.

Idiosyncrasy to cocaine occurs very occasionally; the patient shows signs of sudden collapse and the condition is serious. It must be treated immediately with stimulants, rest and warmth.

Cocaine is never used for injection owing to its toxicity.

Amethocaine (*tetracaine*), *Benoxinate*, *Novesine* and others usually known under proprietary names, are in common use. As they have no mydriatic action they may be used for tonometry.

Common Eye Treatments

They are not under the Misuse of Drugs Act and can conveniently be left out in an emergency 'setting'.

Antiseptic and Antibiotic Drops

These are used in the treatment of infection and also prophylactically. The particular ones in favour at any one time vary widely and the introduction of antibiotics has considerably reduced the use of others.

Penicillin. Its value in ophthalmic work is very considerable. The concentration of the solutions used and the method of application will probably vary with scientific advances. It appears to be specially valuable in cases of acute infection of sudden onset, ophthalmia neonatorum being a typical example. Steroid preparations, such as Predsol and Betnesol are in common use for inflammatory and allergic conditions. *Aureomycin, chloramphenicol, neomycin* and *Soframycin* and other antibiotics are frequently ordered, each drug being effective against particular organisms. When these drugs are used as eye drops they are usually ordered at frequent intervals. For an acute infection penicillin may be instilled every minute for half an hour, followed by every five minutes for half an hour and then at longer intervals. Sensitivity to the drugs may be shown by a skin condition somewhat resembling atropine irritation.

Albucid (sulphacetamide). At the present time this is used in strengths varying from 5–30 per cent.

Examples of silver preparations are *Protargol* and *Argyrol.* If used for a long time they result in argyrosis, an unpleasant staining of the conjunctiva.

Other antiseptics include proflavine 1 in 4,000, zinc chloride or sulphate gr. ½ or gr. 1 to the ounce, and mercurochrome 1–2 per cent.

MISCELLANEOUS DROPS

Adrenaline, 1 in 1,000, is often used as a local vasoconstrictor and is very useful as a haemostatic during operations.

Antistin-Privine drops (antazoline co) are used for allergic conditions. Antistin is an antihistamine and Privine is a vaso-constrictor.

There are a variety of other preparations. The drugs are sometimes combined with an antibiotic.

Common Eye Treatments

Epinephrine 1 *per cent* has been used in open-angle glaucoma to reduce the intra-ocular pressure by decreasing the rate of aqueous production.

Castor Oil, Oleum ricini, is a heavier oil than Paroleine and was generally used as a lubricant by anaesthetists. It can be used as a vehicle for atropine and eserine.

Cod-Liver Oil, Oleum morrhuae, is sometimes used for corneal ulcers.

Paroleine, liquid paraffin, is invaluable for lubrication of the eyeball; three to six drops may be put in at each instillation.

Diagnostic Stains

Fluorescein. This is a stain used for diagnostic purposes. If the corneal epithelium has been injured the area may be invisible until stained with fluorescein when it will show bright green and this is more apparent if the eye is examined with a daylight filter on the lamp. A corneal ulcer takes up the stain with a yellowish green colour, and conjunctival burns are yellow. A usual method in Emergency Departments is to touch the conjunctiva of the lower lid with a glass rod dipped in fluorescein and then wash off the excess stain with normal saline drops.

An alternative method is by the use of narrow strips of filter paper which are prepared by dipping the end in fluorescein solution and dry sterilizing them in a hot-air oven; the application is made by touching the inside of the lower lid with the stained paper and it has the advantage that a minimal amount of stain is used so that it is not necessary to wash away the excess. Fluorescein solution is a good medium for the growth of pathogenic organisms and therefore it should be freshly prepared, and opened bottles should be changed daily.

Rose Bengal, supplied in individual packs, is a diagnostic stain of value in Sjögren's disease.

THE APPLICATION OF OINTMENT

Oculentum is the term for eye ointment. In the local treatment of eyes, ointment is applied to the skin, to the lid margins or inside the lids.

Common Eye Treatments

Applied to the Skin

This is usually for conditions of local inflammation such as that due to atropine irritation when zinc oxide ointment or cream is frequently ordered.

The ointment should be applied from a swab to leave a coating over the inflamed area. A previous application which has become dried can be removed with olive oil.

If mydriatic drops are still being used, it is best to re-apply the ointment before instilling the drop as the coating forms a waterproof protection against further irritation.

N.B. Ointment or oil on the skin renders the lids very difficult to hold for examination or irrigation.

Applied to the Lid Margins

This treatment is ordered for two main purposes; in *Conjunctivitis* it prevents discharge from drying and sealing the lids together. This is more likely to occur at night and will cause much discomfort on waking and also keep the discharge in contact with the eyeball.

The ointment, e.g. boracic, should be applied from a swab along the lash margins, the eye being kept closed during the application.

In *Blepharitis*, inflammation of the lid margins, the ointment must be rubbed well in. The margins will be red and crusted and it is essential that these scabs are completely removed before the antiseptic can be effective. The condition is usually found in children and severe or intractable cases respond very encouragingly to in-patient treatment owing to the difficulty of efficient treatment at home.

To remove the crusts. The patient must be quite comfortable as it takes a little time to carry out the treatment.

It is convenient to use a prepared swab stick moistened with sodium bicarbonate lotion.

For the upper lid, the patient is asked to close his eye and by light pressure the lash margin is slightly everted and scrubbed gently but firmly until all the scabs have been removed. The wool must be changed as required. In bad cases the raw places may bleed a little.

For the lower lid the patient looks up while the lower lid is drawn down.

Common Eye Treatments

When the crusts are removed the ointment can be applied from a swab or a rod, the important point being to massage it well in.

This treatment may be ordered two or three times a day.

Ointment Applied Inside the Lids

When applied in this way the ointment is used as a base for a drug to affect the eye. Its particular advantage over drops is that it remains in the conjunctival sac for a longer time, it acts as a lubricant to the cornea and, for children, it is more likely to be applied effectively at home.

Eye ointment is usually dispensed in a collapsible tube but it may be in a jar to be applied with a glass rod.

Method of application from a tube. This can be easily done and has the advantage that the eye will not be touched with the rod and also the ointment inside the tube cannot be contaminated. The lower lid should be drawn down with a swab, the patient asked to look up and a little stream of ointment is squeezed along the inside of the lid (see plate XV). The end of the tube should not be allowed to touch the lashes; if this accidentally occurs the screw-cap should not be replaced until the nozzle has been wiped on a clean swab and passed through a flame; any ointment in the nozzle that might have been exposed to the heat must be squeezed out on to a swab. For in-patients, a tube must be marked for the particular patient.

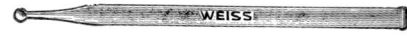

GLASS EYE ROD

Method of application with a glass rod. The rod should be inspected for chips or roughness which would make it unsuitable for use. Some ointment is taken on the end of the rod, a larger amount is taken for a child in case there is difficulty in getting it exactly inside the lid. With a folded swab on the lower lid, it is drawn down and the patient is asked to look up; the rod is placed horizontally inside the lower lid, the patient is asked to close his eye and the rod is withdrawn from the outer side of the eyelids (see plate XIV). If the rod is twisted as it is withdrawn, it will make sure that the ointment is

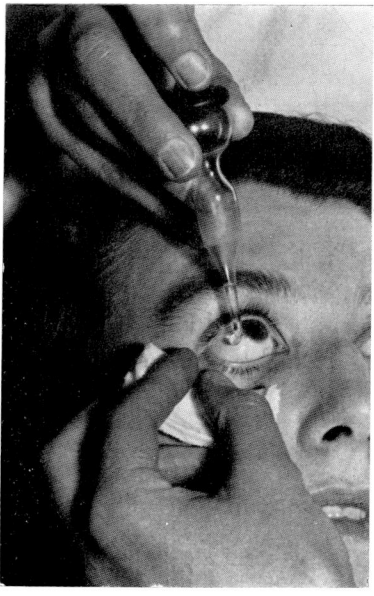
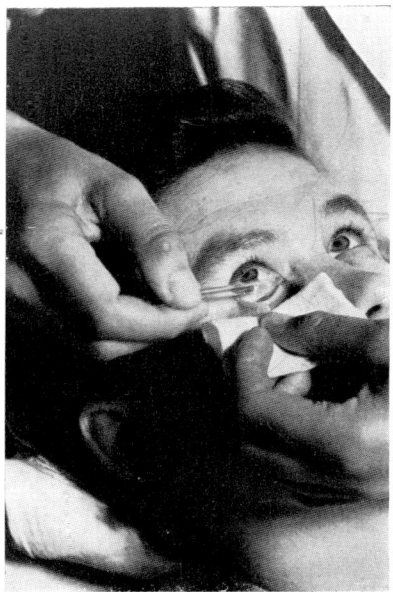

XIII. (above left) Instillation of drops
N.B. The head should be tilted farther back than appears in this photograph

XIV. (above right) Application of ointment with a glass rod

XV. (left) Application of ointment from a tube

XVI. (below) Application of ointment to a baby, using a rod

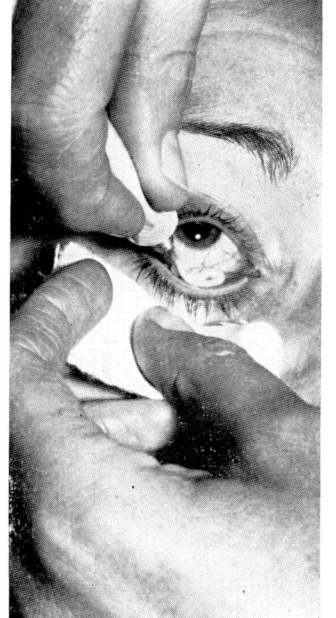
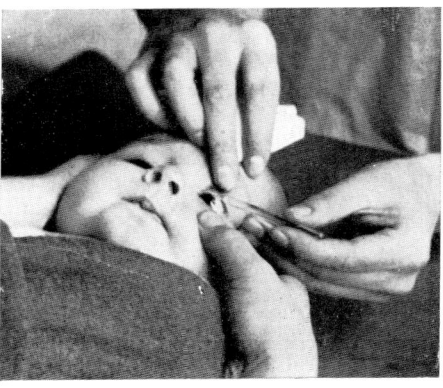

Common Eye Treatments

left inside the lids. The patient should be allowed to open his eye so that it can be seen that the lashes were not rolled in with the ointment.

Possible Difficulties. Children who are resenting treatment or patients with a painful or photophobic eye, may not look up satisfactorily. In this case the upper lid must be controlled with the first finger and the lower one with the second finger on a swab; the ointment should then be put in as swiftly as possible. This is an example of the value of speed; the ointment can often be slipped in during the one instant when the patient chances to be looking up and in any case it will be much less uncomfortable if done quickly (see plate XVI).

Ointment in the Prevention of Symblepharon

Burns of the conjunctiva may result in symblepharon, that is, the adhesion of the lid to the globe, with serious after-effects. This is prevented by passing a rod, covered thickly with ointment, round the upper and lower fornices once or twice daily.

Method. After one instillation of local anaesthetic drops the rod is coated with ointment, half up the stem; the patient is asked to look up while the rod is passed carefully right round the inside of the lower lid. With the patient looking down, a second application is passed round the upper fornix, particular care being taken that it reaches the limits in every part. In this way adhesions which are starting to form are separated and also a layer of ointment is left between the lid and the eyeball.

Notes on Ointments

There is not a large number of ointments in common use. The antibiotic drugs are frequently used, and the particular ones in favour at any time will vary. Steroid drugs are also ordered in the form of ointments and they may be combined with an antibiotic. Because the various proprietary brands are supplied under trade names it is necessary to look carefully at the labels to find the name of the drug in very small print.

Common Eye Treatments

IRRIGATION

The irrigation of an eye is mainly ordered for the purpose of washing the surface of the eyeball and conjunctiva; this is usually required after accidents such as when caustic fluid is splashed in an eye or when dust or lime are showered on the face. In some hospitals an irrigation is part of the routine preparation for operation, being done once in the ward and then again in the theatre. Treatment for conjunctivitis used to include frequent irrigations to wash away discharge but with the use of antibiotics at frequent intervals it is considered better to allow a concentration of the antibiotic to remain in the conjunctival sac.

The aim is a free and copious wash flowing well inside the lids; this can be best obtained if the lotion is non-irritant and at a comfortable temperature and the eyelids gently but firmly controlled.

The Lotion

Normal saline is the lotion most commonly ordered and it is convenient to use autoclaved vacolitres if they are available. Proprietary lotions which contain drugs such as Hazeline, glycerin, adrenaline and rose water are soothing to the eye, but these are not used for irrigation in which a considerable quantity of lotion is required. Boracic lotion was very popular as it can be supplied as crystals to be made up as required; a saturated solution is 4 per cent and therefore it cannot be used in too strong a concentration.

Requisites

In a sterilized pack:
Undine
Small receiver
10 oz. measure jug
10 eye swabs
Small towel
Lotion, bowl of hot water for warming the lotion, protective cape and bag for used swabs.

The lotion, usually normal saline, should be prepared in a jug for use at body temperature. A thermometer may be used but a nurse

Common Eye Treatments

should be able to judge the temperature by pouring a little of the lotion on the inside of her forearm, that being more sensitive than the back of the hand. There is a problem of how to warm the lotion. It may be convenient to stand a vacolitre of sterile saline in a warm water bath, but it is often necessary to put a small jug of lotion in a bowl of hot water. Occasionally the lotion is dispensed in double strength which allows warm water to be added to dilute it.

Undine. This should hold at least four ounces to allow a thorough irrigation. If there is copious discharge it is well to allow for it to be refilled during the treatment. The outflow hole should be large enough for the lotion to flow fairly rapidly, otherwise it is not sufficiently forceful and too tedious for the patient. If the hole is too small it can be enlarged by cutting the spout shorter.

Undine Stand. When autoclave sterilization is not available the undine needs protection when being boiled. An undine stand was used in Eye Hospitals, but a good method is to fill the undine with water and stand it inside the measure jug so that it can be lifted out with the jug. In emergency departments the undine can be kept ready for use in a covered jug.

Lotion Thermometers. These are seldom used owing to the difficulty of sterilization. They were frequently kept in containers of antiseptic lotion and rinsed with tap water but this method is not now considered satisfactory.

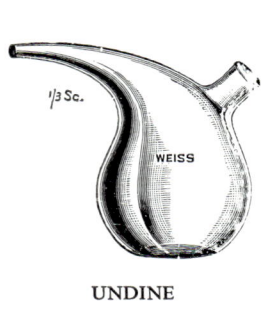

UNDINE

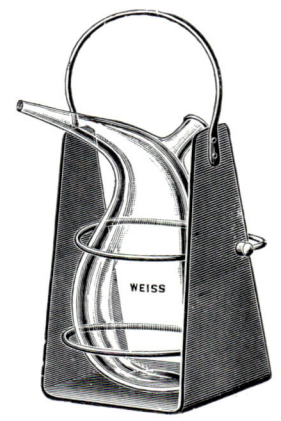

UNDINE STAND

Common Eye Treatments

Irrigation Tray. A light tray which fits the curve of the cheek is ideal. There are special patterns, one being the Fisher's dish. (Mr. Fisher was an Ophthalmic Surgeon.)

A small size kidney receiver with a thin rim can be used very comfortably, but a heavy one is difficult for the patient to hold.

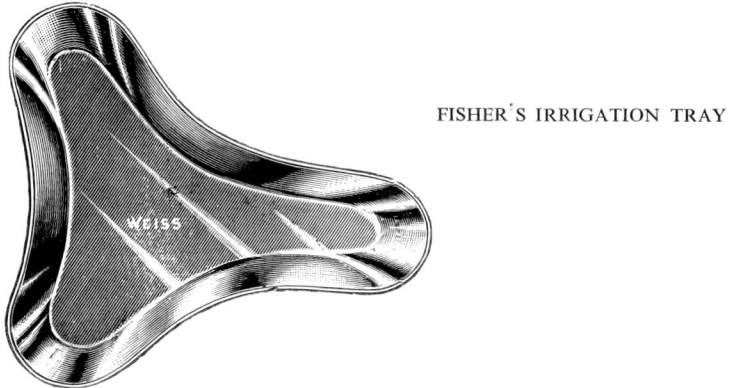

FISHER'S IRRIGATION TRAY

Mackintosh Cape. This is essential and it must be large enough to cover the shoulder, or shoulder and pillow. It should always be *tied* round the neck in such a way that it will protect the patient should there be a spill.

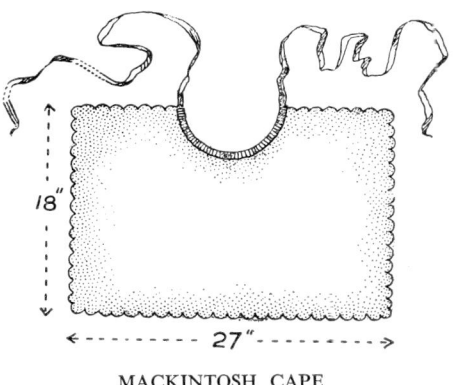

MACKINTOSH CAPE

Common Eye Treatments

Bowl of Swabs.
Small receiver or bag for used Swabs.

Position of the Patient

The patient may be in bed or in a chair with a head rest. The head must be comfortably supported with the chin almost horizontal and the head inclined to the side of the eye to be treated.

Two common faults are:

The head is not held sufficiently back so that the lotion flows on to the cheek and into the eye, or the head is inclined to the opposite side, in which case the used lotion will run down the side of the nose instead of into the tray.

It is never advisable to attempt an irrigation with the patient sitting in a chair without a head rest; he will be most uncomfortable trying to keep his head back which, in fact, he cannot do satisfactorily.

For an in-patient who is dressed in the ward, a pillow and rug can be arranged so that he lies with his head at the foot end of the bed. This is very convenient for the nurse.

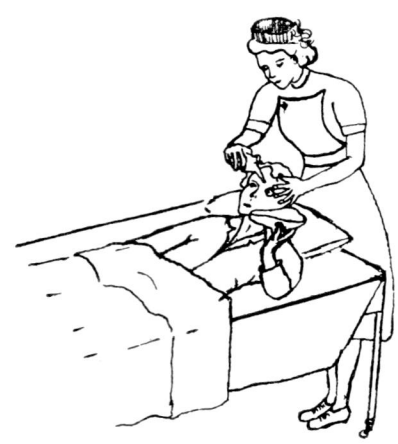

PATIENT LYING WITH HEAD AT FOOT OF BED FOR IRRIGATION

Common Eye Treatments

Where to stand when irrigating. The usual practice is for the nurse to stand behind the chair or end of the bed.

It is not wrong to stand on the side of the eye to be treated, facing the patient's head: it may be necessary to use this position if the bed may not be moved or if the nurse is not tall enough to reach over the top of the bed.

As with all eye treatments it is essential that the light should be adequate. The patient facing a window or light is satisfactory.

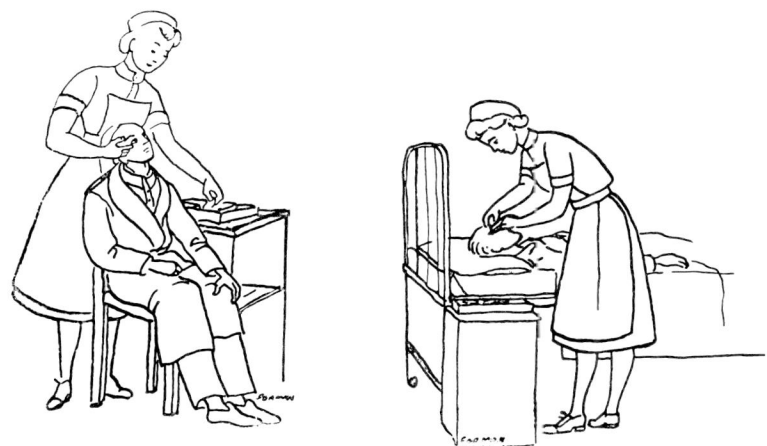

NURSE STANDING BEHIND CHAIR AND AT SIDE OF BED

METHOD OF IRRIGATING (see plates XVII, XVIII, XIX)

1. If there is much discharge this must be removed with moist swabs.

2. If ointment or oily drops have been applied they should be removed from the lids as far as possible: greasy lids are difficult to hold open.

3. The patient's head should be comfortably settled and he be given the tray to hold pressed against his cheek (never under the chin). He is responsible for keeping it close to his face, but he cannot see if it is level and that is the nurse's care.

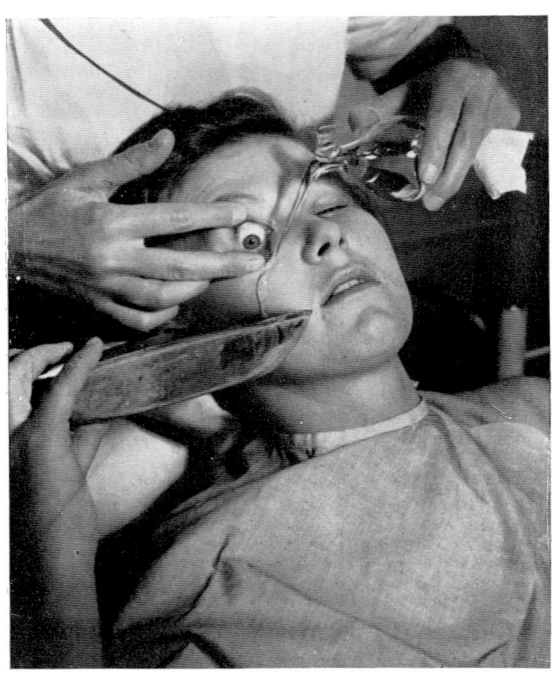

XVII. Irrigation: the flow of lotion started on the cheek

IRRIGATION OF THE EYE

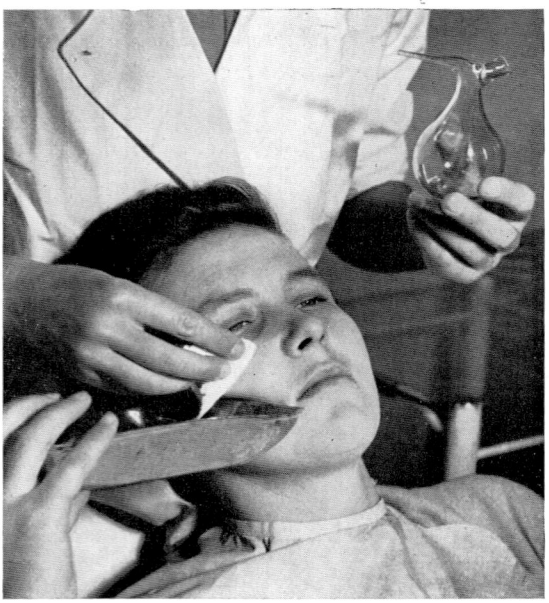

XVIII. Irrigation: the cheek dried before the undine is put down

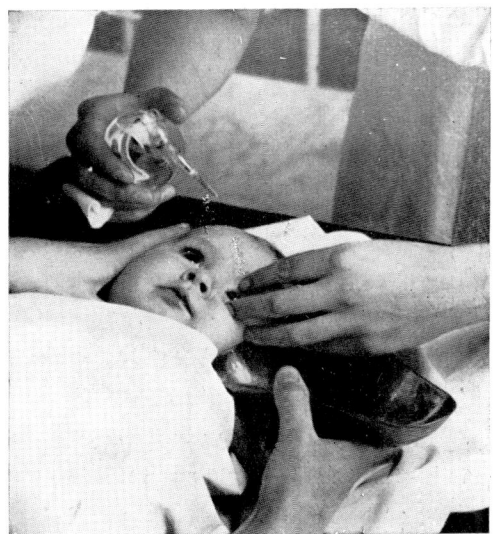

XIX. Irrigation for a baby

4. The undine is held in the left hand *for the right eye* and a swab is tucked between the third and fourth fingers so that it is ready when required.

5. The lids are held apart with the first and second fingers of the right hand, the tip of the finger being placed near to the lashes and the loose skin drawn gently down and then held firmly against the orbital ridge. When taking the upper lid care must be taken not to press on the eyeball as that is always uncomfortable and if the eye is tender it is acutely painful. No patient can hold his lids open during an irrigation, and it is much easier for him to feel that they are securely held. When they are opened the patient should be asked to open his other eye as both relax together. Should a lid slip from the finger during the irrigation another grip can be taken without stopping the flow.

6. The patient is warned that the lotion is coming and it is poured on to his cheek first so that he can feel the temperature; if that is comfortable it is brought up to the nasal side of the eye.

Common Eye Treatments

7. The undine should be held about an inch away from the lids: if too close the lids may be touched and if too far away the pressure is too high.

Once the flow is started it should be kept constant by holding the undine tipped fully; it cannot flow too fast and intermittent trickles are most irritating to the patient. It is usual to keep the flow directed over the inner canthus and to ask the patient to look up and down and to the sides, thereby washing the whole of the eyeball. Special care should be taken to draw down the lower lid with the patient looking up and irrigate thoroughly into the lower fornix.

It is surprising how much it helps the patient if he is talked to during the treatment; instructed where to look; asked to open the other eye; assured that he is doing well, and told when the treatment is nearly finished.

8. When the undine is empty, *and before it is put down*, the swab from the left hand is taken by the right and the lids are quickly dried, also the cheek down to the edge of the tray; then the tray is taken from the patient and that and the undine are put down. (If the tray is taken first, lotion will trickle down the neck, and if the nurse turns to put down the undine first the patient thinks that all is over and is likely to sit forward and spill the contents of the tray.) Another swab is taken immediately to complete the drying and remove any discharge.

It may be necessary to irrigate an everted upper lid, e.g. after painting with silver nitrate. It is convenient to evert it with one hand, but it is quite simple to use a glass rod which can be dropped into the tray held by the patient, after which the undine can be picked up.

Common difficulties and reasons for failure

1. The patient screws his eye tightly and it cannot be held open. This may be due to discomfort from the following causes:

    The lotion is too hot or too cold.
    The lotion is stinging the eye.
    Pressure on the eyeball causes him pain.
    He feels lotion escaping down his neck.
    He is frightened or is a child.

After attention to the particular point at fault, it is best to ask

Common Eye Treatments

the patient to concentrate his attention on opening the other eye and then, gently but firmly, to do the treatment as quickly as possible.

2. Lids which are slippery with ointment cannot always be held properly, and it is best to be certain that the head is well back so that the lotion will flow in even if the lids are not well open.

3. Lids are tender, e.g. with a stye; in this case the unaffected lid only should be held.

4. The flow from the undine is so slow that it does not effectively wash away the discharge and the patient tires because it takes too long; the remedy is to make the outflow hole larger.

5. The patient is unable to hold the tray satisfactorily against his cheek. Children are not able to do so and often the patient is too deaf to follow the instructions. Whatever the cause, it is best to get an assistant.

6. A patient, especially a baby, may have so much oedema of the lids that it is impossible to separate them or to see the eyeball. It is unwise for a nurse to use lid retractors and she must inform the surgeon of her difficulty. The fact of giving a small baby something to suck will often cause him to open his eye.

Irrigation With Other Apparatus

From a Douche Can or similar container; from Wool Swabs or with an Eye Bath.

Douche Can. The apparatus is fitted with tubing, regulating clip and irrigation nozzle. Such equipment was provided in Gas Decontamination Centres; it was certainly practical for this purpose as an unlimited supply of lotion could be used for each treatment and many patients could be dealt with very rapidly. For general use the temperature of the lotion is difficult to regulate and the apparatus is cumbersome to sterilize and to store.

Wool Swabs. For the irrigation of a baby at home or of a patient for himself, a fairly satisfactory washout can be obtained by using warmed lotion from a bowl and squeezing it into the eye from a *large* piece of wool. The adult can hold his head over a basin: for an infant the problem is how to catch the used lotion:

(*a*) A large piece of absorbent material can be held to the cheek. This is convenient but extravagant.

Common Eye Treatments

(*b*) The baby's head can be held over a bucket.

(*c*) There is a method of using a marine sponge and squeezing it out. This is easy but obviously not to be recommended owing to the difficulty of, and risk of inadequate, cleansing of the sponge.

Eye Bath. It is argued that an eye bath is useless because it provides no flow of lotion washing the eye. It is certainly inadequate if there is discharge to be removed, but it is so simple and easy to use on oneself, besides being economical of lotion, that it seems worth allowing it. Methods in the home which require cups, bowls, basins and towels are a greater source of infection and the treatment is less likely to be carried out thoroughly and regularly. The eye bath should be well washed before use: it should be filled two-thirds full with warmed lotion: the head must be bent forward and the bath fitted over the eye: then the head is bent back so that the lotion enters the eye as the lids are opened and shut and the eye moved about.

This method is particularly satisfactory for eyes which have been irritated with fumes or for chronic conjunctivitis, but is must be stressed that there is no beneficial washing away of discharge.

3

EYE TREATMENTS (continued)

THE APPLICATION OF HEAT

Heat is applied locally to the eye to increase the blood supply, to relieve pain, or to hasten the absorption of drugs. There is no doubt that patients appreciate the benefit of heat.

The usual method of application of moist heat is by hot bathing; dry heat can be applied by an electric eye warmer or by electrotherapy: the latter treatment is carried out by trained electrotherapists; if it is being used in conjunction with moist heat, it is inadvisable to give a hot bathing within two hours of the electrical treatment.

HOT SPOON BATHING

The aim is to steam the eye rather than to bathe it with warm water (see plate XXI).

Requisites

Bowl, or jug, holding at least 2 pints of *boiling* water.
Padded wooden spoon.
Mackintosh cape.
Small bowl of swabs and a receiver for used ones.

The wooden spoon can be padded with any absorbent material. The padding should be on the back and over the end. If old linen is used as a covering, the pieces can be boiled and used again unless pus is present, e.g. with a stye. A rubber band to hold the linen in position can be left on the handle and boiled with the spoon after use.

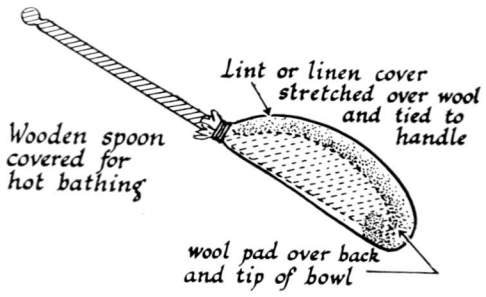

COVERED WOODEN SPOON

The patient should be comfortably seated at a table or supported in bed in such a way that there is no risk of the bowl being upset.

The mackintosh cape will prevent his clothes becoming damp with the steam (see plate XXI).

Instructions to the patient:
1. To keep his eye closed.
2. To keep his head well over the bowl and the padded side of the spoon near to the eye; the steam is more beneficial than contact with the hot spoon.
3. To continue for about five or ten minutes. Longer than this makes the skin soft and is very tiring to the patient.

The treatment can be repeated two to four-hourly as required.

STEAM BATHING (see plates XX and XXII)
The following is an alternative to Hot Spoon Bathing as a method of applying moist heat to an eye. The instruction card can be given to patients who have to carry it out at home.

'*Steam Bathing an Eye*
Fill a jug, 1 pint–2 pint size, three-quarters full of boiling water. Sit at a table with the jug in front of you and *let the steam from the boiling water warm your eye* by holding that side of your face a short distance away from the jug. *It is important to keep your eye closed all the time.*

Continue the treatment for five to ten minutes.'

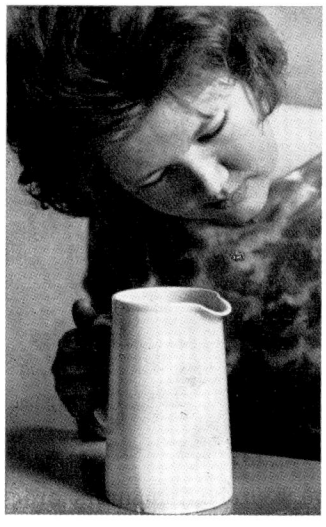 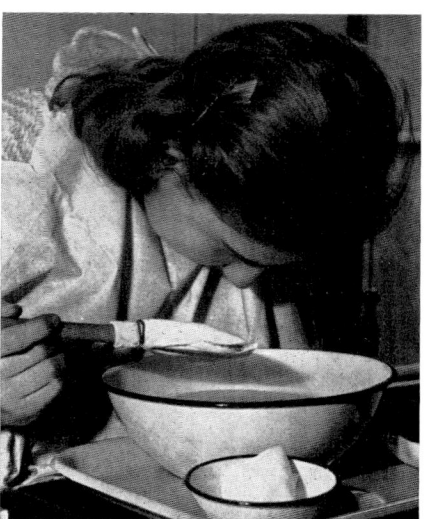

XX. Steam bathing an eye as an alternative to hot spoon bathing

XXI. Hot Spoon Bathing

XXII. Steam Bathing an Eye

Fill a jug, 1–2 pint size, three-quarters full of boiling water. Sit at a table with the jug in front of you and *let the steam from the boiling water warm your eye* by holding that side of your face a short distance away from the jug. It is important to keep your eye closed all the time. Continue the treatment for 5–10 minutes.

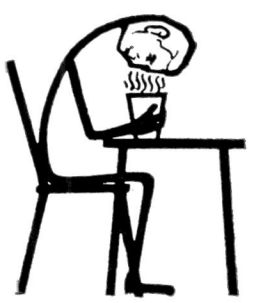

It is preferable to use a china jug rather than a stainless steel one so that the handle can be held.

The advantages of the above treatment are:

Eye Treatments

1. It gives a very comfortable feeling of warmth and does not involve any pressure on an eye which is painful.

2. The temperature can be easily controlled by the distance at which the head is held from the top of the jug.

3. There is no risk of contaminating a wooden spoon used for cooking and no possibility of damp padding on the spoon being used several times for the sake of economy.

4. Because it is easy to find a jug or similar receptacle at home, it is more likely that the treatment will be carried out regularly.

If *drops* or *ointment* are ordered with hot bathing they should be instilled beforehand as the heat will aid their absorption, e.g. atropine or eserine. If immediate effect is required, more drops can be put in during the bathing: this is often done in an out-patient department. On the other hand, the heat might detract from the effect of the drug, e.g. penicillin, and in this case it should be put in afterwards. Strictly speaking, the treatment ought to be done in the order in which it is written on the treatment card.

Hot Bathing for a Child. This cannot be carried out with a spoon. The only effective method is for the nurse to foment the eye continuously for ten minutes at a time. Circles of gamgee make convenient fomentations which should be started warm, the heat being increased as the child gets accustomed to it.

Hot Fomentations are occasionally ordered, but owing to their small size they are useless if applied singly and the more practical way is to foment for a short time and then leave a warm dry pad over the eye.

DRY HEAT

The electric eye warmer has a flat piece containing the element which is placed in the middle of the wool of an eye pad and then bandaged on to the eye.

The flex should be held by a turn of the bandage so that movement of the patient will not drag on the pad. It is more comfortable if the flex is separated from the forehead by a layer of bandage which means putting it in the second turn. It is very important to bandage the pad firmly enough to keep it close to the eye. A large pad of wool over the eye pad helps to keep the warmth in.

The warmer should be adjusted to feel comfortably warm to the

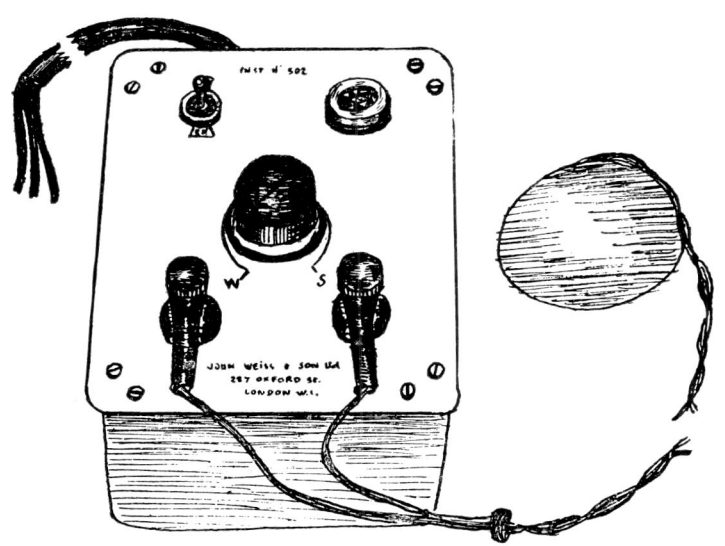

ELECTRIC EYE WARMER

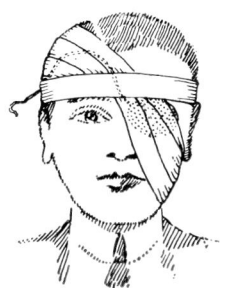

EYE WARMER BANDAGED IN POSITION

patient and if he is intelligent he can be shown how to adjust it for himself. It is impossible to keep it set at the same point as there is a slight difference in the amount of wool separating it from the eye with each application. If the patient has much pain he may not feel

Eye Treatments

excessive heat and in this case should not be allowed to increase it for himself.

It can be left on for twenty minutes to half an hour at a time, as frequently as required.

This method of applying heat has the great advantage of causing the minimum of disturbance to the patient.

A Rubber Hot-Water Bottle can be used to provide local heat. It should not be filled more than half full so that it is soft to lie on: the temperature of the water should be about 130° F and two covers may be put on the bottle.

THE APPLICATION OF COLD

This may be used to reduce congestion or arrest haemorrhage. Ice bathing, Cold Compresses or Ice Poultice may be ordered. A very effective method is for the nurse to sit by the patient and apply iced compresses continuously for ten minutes at a time. The rhythmic changing is very soothing.

THE CUTTING OF EYE-LASHES

Eye-lashes are usually cut in preparation for operation: it reduces the risk of infection and makes the subsequent dressing easier.

Patients should be assured that lashes will grow to a normal length in a few weeks. If there is a tendency for the lower lid to turn in, it is better not to cut the lower lashes as they would be more irritating as they grow again. Some surgeons, who use a guarded speculum, prefer that only the lashes on the outer third of the lids should be cut. If a patient has a strong objection to having the lashes cut it is often wise to leave it to the discretion of the surgeon.

Requisites. Sharp, blunt-pointed scissors: either Conjunctival scissors or Surgical ones, but not Stitch scissors. Vaseline Petroleum Jelly, Swabs and Receiver.

Method. It is essential that the patient be in a good light with his head comfortably supported.

The blades of the scissors should be smeared with Vaseline Petroleum Jelly which will cause the cut lashes to adhere to them:

Eye Treatments

if a little Vaseline Petroleum Jelly is left inside the folded swab it can be reapplied as required.

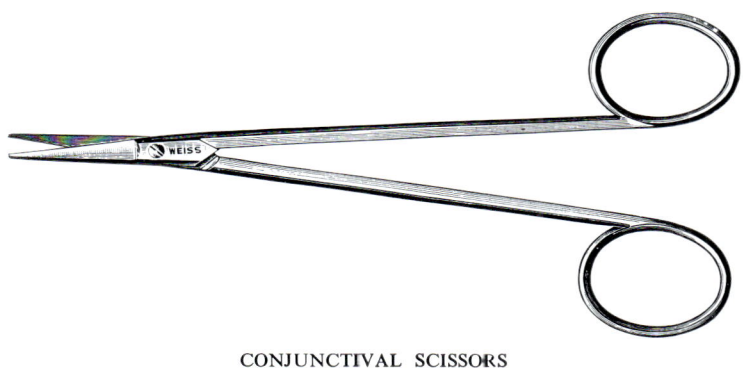

CONJUNCTIVAL SCISSORS

The eye should be kept closed for the upper lid and if the lid margin is slightly everted it is easier to slip the scissors under the lashes. For the lower lid the patient is asked to look up. The lashes should be cut fairly short, but it is not of serious consequence if they are not cut down to the edge of the lid.

The right eye is easier because, with the scissors held in the right hand, cutting is towards the nose. For the left eye it is better to stand to the side of the patient.

Possible mistakes are:

Lashes being allowed to fall into the eye and remaining as foreign bodies.

The skin of the lid may be snipped; this sounds very careless, but it can occur with a child who moves suddenly.

The lashes may be cut unevenly with a few long ones left at the ends.

It must be stressed that it is impossible to cut lashes without a good light and suitable scissors. If a child is frightened it is quite reasonable to leave it until the patient is in the theatre when the eye is cocainized or a general anaesthetic has been given.

Eye Treatments

EPILATION OF EYE-LASHES

Trichiasis is the condition of ingrowing eye-lashes with resulting irritation of the cornea. It is usually due to chronic disease of the lids and radical treatment is very difficult. The irritation causes corneal ulceration with serious scarring which permanently affects the eyesight: besides this risk, it causes intense discomfort and the lashes have to be removed. This can be done by epilation, the pulling out of lashes, or by electrolysis which destroys the root of the lash. The latter treatment affords permanent relief, but is only possible if there are not a large number to be dealt with.

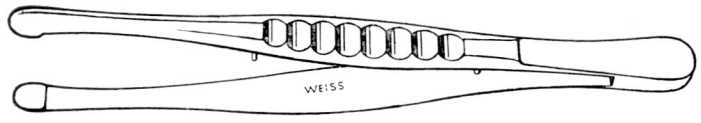

EPILATION FORCEPS

Method (see plate XXIII). This is not a painful procedure, in fact, it is welcomed for the relief given. Epilation forceps are of various patterns, but all have blunt tips to allow a firm grip to be taken on the lash.

It is essential to have a specially good light and a corneal loupe should be worn; this may not always seem necessary, but diseased lashes are very fine and white and can only be seen under magnification. If a nurse does not accustom herself to the use of a loupe she will miss these fine lashes.

The lid should be slightly everted with a swab held under the finger so that the forceps can be wiped on it to remove each lash. The lash should be gripped firmly near to its base and be pulled out sharply; these lashes are brittle and if the top is broken off it will be impossible to grip the remaining stump.

The fine lashes are extremely difficult to see and often require a dark background of cornea to show them up: it is poor work if a single ingrowing lash is left.

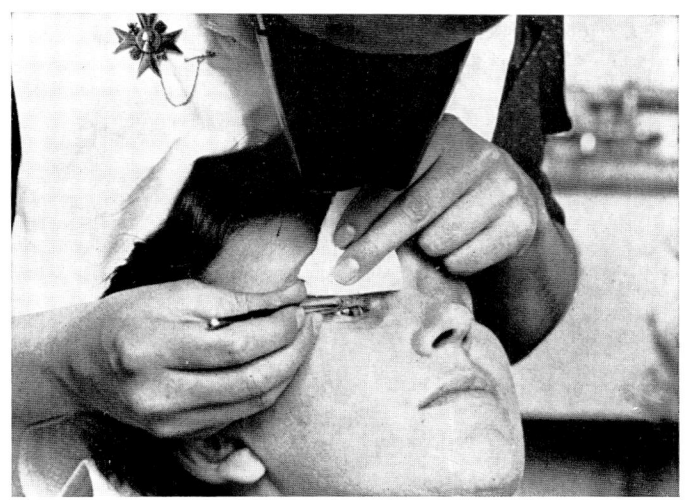

XXIII. Epilation of lashes

At intervals the lid must be allowed to lie in its normal position to show which lashes are actually touching the eyeball.

Unfortunately they grow again in a few weeks and the treatment may have to be repeated for years.

APPLICATIONS TO THE CONJUNCTIVA

PAINTING THE CONJUNCTIVA

The conjunctival surface of the lids may be painted with various antiseptics such as silver nitrate, 1 or 2 per cent, or penicillin.

Requisites. Silver nitrate or other drug (gr. 5 to the fluid ounce equals 1 per cent).

Watch glass or pannikin.

Prepared swab sticks.

Swabs and Receiver.

After silver nitrate it is usual to irrigate with saline as the silver causes a coagulation of the surface and the tiny shreds can be washed away.

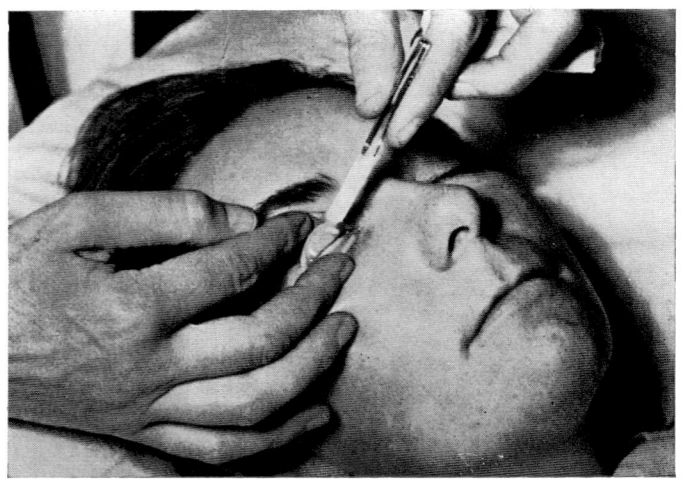

XXIV. Painting the conjunctiva with Silver Nitrate

Method (see plate XXIV). The swab stick is moistened with silver nitrate and a swab tucked between the fingers of the left hand: the lids are everted, using one hand or the uncovered end of the stick: the patient is then asked to close his eye tightly and this brings the everted lids together over the cornea. The solution should be dabbed freely on the conjunctiva, the excess being absorbed with a swab before the lids are allowed to turn back. The lids must be everted again during the irrigation when tiny greyish shreds will be seen to wash away.

It is not wrong to evert the upper and lower lids separately and paint them one at a time.

Silver nitrate stings the eye and it is more comfortable to put in one drop of cocaine before using the 2 per cent solution. The silver nitrate stick is *never* used for this purpose being much too caustic.

Copper Sulphate Application. Copper stick is ordered for the conjunctival granulations which occur in trachoma. The first few applications are intensely painful and the eye should be cocainized. The

Eye Treatments

lid is everted and the copper stick rubbed firmly on the follicles. A drop of Paroleine helps to relieve the subsequent discomfort.

LAMELLAE

These are very thin gelatin discs containing a drug, e.g. hyoscine or penicillin; they are applied by being placed inside the lower lid.

Their advantage is that none of the drug can fall on to the skin as with drops or ointment and this reduces the skin irritation sometimes occurring with the use of mydriatics. Instructions, provided with lamellae, advise the application by means of a small camel hair brush. Brushes are very difficult to sterilize satisfactorily and the lamellae can be picked up by touching it with a damp glass rod.

INSUFFLATION OF POWDER

This is rarely ordered at the present time; an example is calomel powder in the treatment of corneal ulcer. An insufflator may be used; the powder must be shaken down to the tip of it and it is then held about an inch away from the separated eyelids and the powder insufflated on to the cornea.

The insufflator and the powder must be quite dry to ensure an even spray.

STRAPPING OF LIDS FOR ENTROPION

Entropion is the turning in of the lid margin, resulting in the lashes lying against the eyeball. It may be caused by injury to or disease of the lids; in the elderly it can be due to spasm of the orbicularis muscle. It must be corrected owing to the irritation caused by the lashes.

It is much more frequent in the lower lid and a simple treatment is the strapping of the lid. A small length of half-inch adhesive strapping is cut with the upper edge rounded to prevent corners touching the eyeball. The upper edge should be pressed on to the skin as close to the lashes as possible and a pleat of skin is made under the strapping so that the lid is drawn down. After it is applied the patient should be asked to squeeze his eye shut so that it can be seen if the strapping is still effective in holding the lid out. The disadvantages

Eye Treatments

are that tears may loosen the strapping, and in any case it soon gets soiled and looks unpleasant on the cheek. The patient can be taught to reapply it for himself.

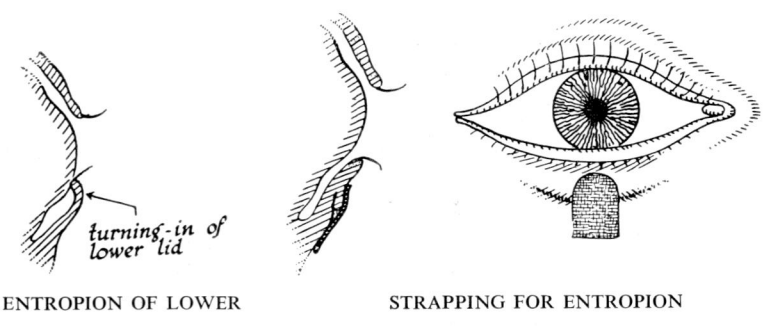

ENTROPION OF LOWER LID

STRAPPING FOR ENTROPION

Further measures include a stitch through the lid so that the silk can be strapped to the cheek or a plastic operation on the lid may be performed.

EXPRESSION OF THE LACHRYMAL SAC

It is comparatively common for infants to suffer from blocked lachrymal apparatus resulting in a watering, and, probably, a discharging eye.

The treatment includes swabbing the eye clean and instilling drops into the nasal corner, but this is more effective if the mother is taught to express the sac to empty it of discharge before using the drops.

The baby's lower lid should be drawn down to expose the punctum; the tip of the finger is then pressed on the side of the nose over the sac. Firm pressure will empty the sac so that a bead of discharge appears at the punctum. It is hoped that the antiseptic drops will then run down into the sac.

The mother should be taught to express the sac each time she feeds the baby. The cure will not be spectacular, but it is rare for the condition not to clear up completely and the mother can be reassured.

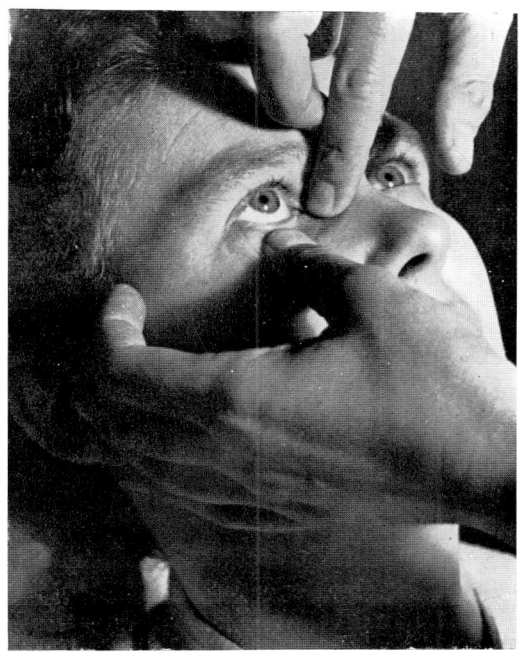

XXV. Expression of Lachrymal Sac

The method is the same for adults: it is easier owing to the larger size of the structures (see plate XXV).

THE CARE OF AN INSENSITIVE EYE

Interference with the sensory nerve to the eye will cause the surface of the eye to become insensitive. The danger is that the lids will not close reflexly to any irritant and the cornea may become damaged without the knowledge of the patient. Very serious corneal ulcers and scarring, with loss of vision, may result.

The treatment aims at keeping the surface of the eye constantly lubricated and the cornea protected from injury. A dry pad and bandage should be avoided in all circumstances as the eye may open underneath and the cornea will become rubbed.

Eye Treatments

The lubricant may be oily drops or ointment; whatever is used must be applied very generously so that the surface of the eye is kept moist.

In cases of corneal ulceration a covering may be necessary. This can take the form of Tulle Gras inside a pad or a pad spread *thickly* with sterile ointment. Some surgeons will not risk any pad and prefer a lubricant and shade. Whatever the treatment the nurse must appreciate the danger and be certain that nothing dry can touch the cornea.

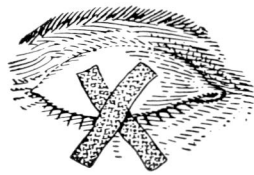

LIDS STRAPPED CLOSED

Strapping the Lids. In certain cases the lids may be strapped closed. Two pieces of half-inch strappings are applied and left for a few days; one disadvantage is that the lids and lashes are very difficult to clean afterwards. The strapping should be covered by a pad and bandage. In advanced cases a Tarsorrhaphy may be performed, the lid margins being stitched together over the eyeball.

The condition of corneal exposure must be similarly treated when due to facial paralysis, exophthalmos or deep coma: in the latter condition the eyes remain open and the corneae will become dry and may ulcerate very rapidly. Operations on the lids may leave the cornea temporarily exposed and the same care is needed. There are protective side-pieces available to clip on to glasses.

4

INVESTIGATIONS, TREATMENTS AND MINOR SURGERY

The following investigations and treatments are frequently carried out in an eye clinic. A general trained nurse would not be expected to undertake them unless she had had special experience, but she should know how to prepare for them.

SYRINGING OF LACHRYMAL SAC (see plate XXVI)

This is carried out for investigation of epiphora, a 'watering eye', in treatment of lachrymal obstruction and by some surgeons as a routine preparation for cataract operation.

Requisites. A special syringe with a luer fitting cannula can be used, but when equipment is prepared by a Central Sterile Supplies Department Service, it is convenient to use the same cannula on a 2 ml. disposable syringe.

Two dilators and cannulae should be provided if there is obvious infection and both sides are to be syringed.

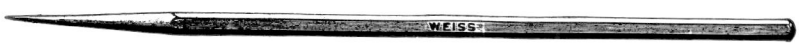

PUNCTUM DILATOR

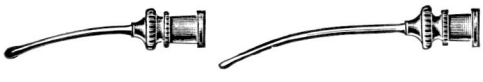

LACHRYMAL SAC CANNULA

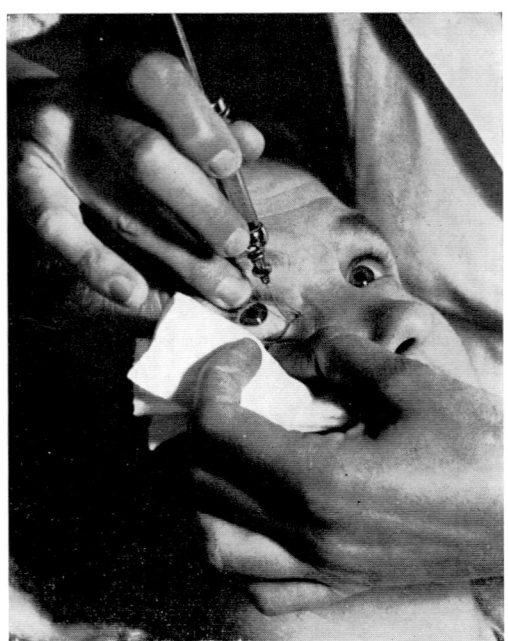

XXVI. Syringing of Lachrymal Sac: insertion of the cannula

The fluid can be water but one with a distinctive taste, such as saline, is of value if the patency is doubtful. A drop of fluorescein added to the fluid will colour the saliva and also help in doubtful cases. Unless there is infection, the patient can be told to swallow the liquid.

Some surgeons like a drop of local anaesthetic instilled just before commencing.

A probe may be required, in which case, a set of fairly fine probes, numbers 0000 and 000, 00 and 0, and 1 and 2 will be necessary. He may need Novocain to syringe into the sac and sterile paraffin for lubrication of the probe.

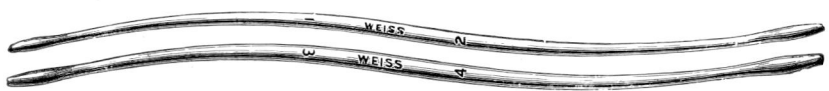

LACHRYMAL PROBE

Investigations, Treatments and Minor Surgery

Infants' sacs are difficult to syringe and a brief general anaesthetic may be required.

If a nurse is doing the syringing, the following points should be noted:

1. The patient can be told that the watering of his eye may be due to a blocked tear duct and it is intended to syringe it with a little salt water which should pass into his throat and can be swallowed.

2. Two swabs should be held on the lid so that if the fluid returns it will not trickle down the cheek.

3. There may be difficulty in inserting the cannula into a small punctum: this is assisted by a drop of local anaesthetic, more thorough dilatation and the stretching of the canaliculus by drawing the lid to the outer side away from the nose.

Occasionally the surgeon's help must be sought.

4. If the sac is not patent, the fluid may return through the upper punctum.

5. If the sac is not patent, *pressure must not be used* as it might force the fluid into the surrounding tissues with resulting cellulitis.

6. The result should be reported as, 'freely patent', or the degree of obstruction stated, as the case may be.

The cannulae must be looked after for blockage or bending. An unobservant nurse can confuse them with hypodermic needles even sending them to be sharpened.

BACTERIOLOGICAL CULTURE OF THE CONJUNCTIVAL SAC

A swab from the lower conjunctival sac is cultured for twenty-four to forty-eight hours. This is a routine precaution before intra-ocular operations except in emergencies: swabs are also taken for diagnostic purposes in cases of infection.

Antiseptic treatment must be discontinued for a clear twenty-four hours before the culture is taken.

The taking of the material for culture is often done by the bacteriologist in the laboratory and this is considered to be the most satisfactory. If a nurse is required to take it the following points are of importance:

1. It is best for the material to be taken on a platinum loop which

Investigations, Treatments and Minor Surgery

has been sterilized by passing it through the flame of a spirit lamp. The loop is passed along the lower fornix and the material should be transferred straight on to an agar plate which is sent to the laboratory as soon as possible. In some hospitals the test is done using a sterilized throat swab; the swab stick is put back into the sterile test tube and taken to the laboratory where it is plated out.

2. If the lachrymal sac is expressed (see plate XXV) before the test is done any infection in the sac will be collected on the loop. Both lids should be controlled and, with the patient looking up, the loop is passed along the lower fornix.

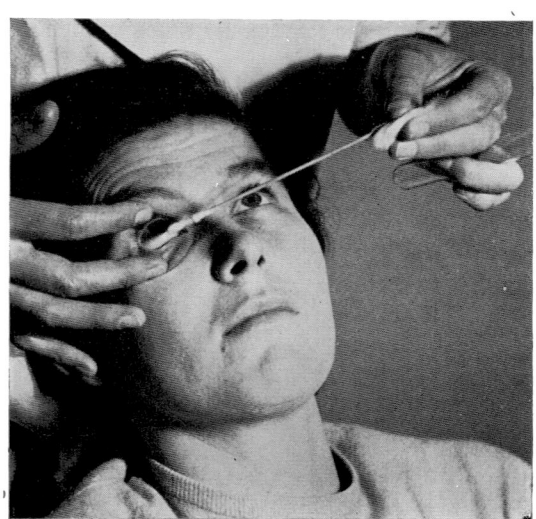

XXVII. The taking of a conjunctival swab for culture

3. It will be found convenient if the culture plates or the tubes containing the throat swabs are labelled for right and left eye before the swabs are taken.

Results of the Culture. If the result is doubtful the bacteriologist may require forty-eight hours. Pneumococci are particularly serious and may be present in a healthy looking eye. They sometimes come from the lachrymal sac.

Investigations, Treatments and Minor Surgery

The number of bacteria varies from a single colony to a heavy growth. With the rapid advances in bacteriology new types are constantly being found and their sensitivity to specific drugs is of great importance.

REMOVAL OF SUTURES

Conjunctival sutures are usually of black silk, but dyed silk may be used to distinguish particular ones, as in a ptosis operation. If catgut is used it will be left to absorb unless it is acting as an irritant.

Conjunctiva unites rapidly and stitches are removed after about four days. In squint operations, the stitches may be through muscles as well as conjunctiva, and these must not be taken out without special instructions. Some surgeons do not tie conjunctival sutures but leave them as a running thread; these can easily be removed by taking the end with forceps and drawing the stitch out.

The removal of *corneal* and *corneo-scleral sutures* requires particular skill and it is usually done by the surgeon or an experienced sister.

Requisites for Removal of Sutures.

Stitch scissors, suture forceps and speculum in a tray.

Bowl of swabs.

Sterile towel.

Cocaine or other local anaesthetic drops.

The eye must be well cocainized and the patient arranged comfortably with a good light.

Possible difficulties. This procedure does not often present difficulty unless the patient is very nervous and unco-operative; if the eye is not kept still the forceps holding the stitch will pull on the eye and cause pain however well it has been cocainized.

Children like being told that 'it is only unpicking'. They sometimes require a brief anaesthetic.

If the stitches are far back from the cornea, as after trephining or some operations for retinal detachment, it can be difficult to pick up the stitch unless the patient looks very far in the opposite direction: the use of a lid retractor instead of a speculum, or an assistant to hold the lids, will allow them to be picked up more easily.

Pink or pale coloured silk can be hard to see on the conjunctiva.

Investigations, Treatments and Minor Surgery

If there is swelling of the tissues and the stitches have been tied tightly, as in some squint operations, they may be almost buried and it can be impossible to see where to cut the knot. It may be advisable to ask permission to leave them for a few days.

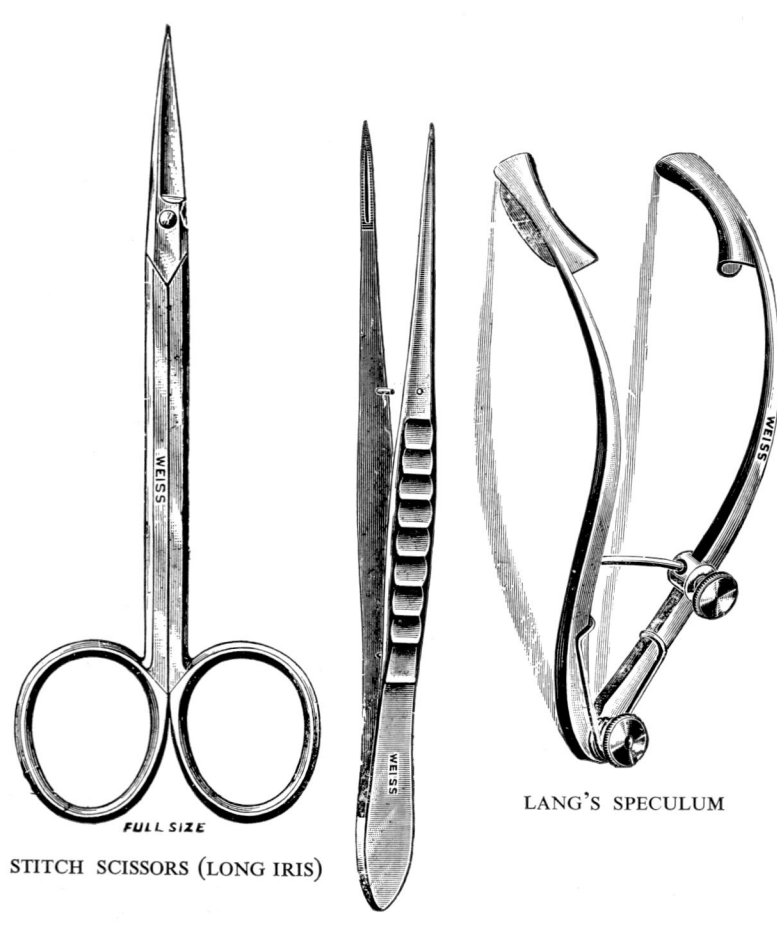

STITCH SCISSORS (LONG IRIS)

LANG'S SPECULUM

SUTURE FORCEPS: MOORFIELD'S PATTERN

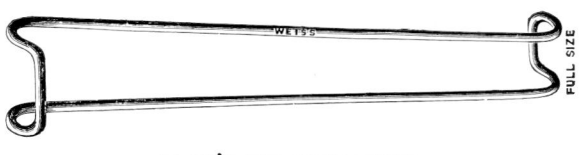

LANG'S LID RETRACTOR

REMOVAL OF CORNEAL FOREIGN BODY

This is a common form of injury and it must be dealt with as soon as possible, or it will irritate and infect the cornea. It may be so small that it can only be seen under magnification. If the foreign body has blown into the eye it will be superficial and can often be removed with a damp swab after a drop of Decicain has been instilled. If it does not come away readily more damage will be done with a swab than with a needle.

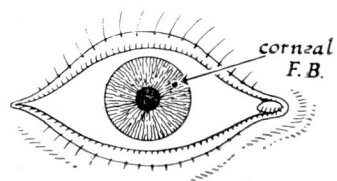

CORNEAL FOREIGN BODY

Corneal foreign bodies usually result from grinding or work where there are minute flying particles, and these may become deeply embedded in the cornea. If they are of metal they will quickly cause rusting of the surrounding cornea.

Instruments used for removing corneal foreign bodies

A *capsulotomy needle*, e.g. a *Beer's needle*, is frequently used. This instrument has a sharp point and a cutting edge extending a few millimetres from the point which makes it effective for removing the rust ring which occurs when a metallic speck has been lying on the moist corneal surface. These needles require skilful sharpening and are usually posted to ophthalmic instrument makers for the purpose.

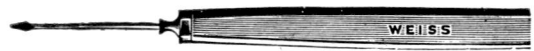

BEER'S NEEDLE

Cluckie's foreign body instrument consists of a metal handle supplied with detachable points which are disposable, but they are not quite so good as the capsulotomy needles.

A *spud* has a blunt end and used to be considered a safer instrument in less experienced hands, but its use causes more damage to the corneal epithelium, and it is less effective for removing the foreign bodies.

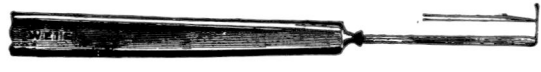

SPUD

A *hypodermic needle* can be used, and the disposable types are very satisfactory.

Requisites. Foreign body needle, local anaesthetic drops, swabs and a corneal loupe. A good light is essential.

Unless the eye is inflamed, two or three instillations of drops are sufficient. A speculum is not used as the movement of the upper lid over the cornea is useful during the removal.

The foreign body is usually fairly easy to deal with, but the rust ring may be very difficult, or impossible, to remove completely on the first occasion.

The patient is often reluctant to have his eye covered as the anaesthetic will render it painless and he feels that it is cured; he should be told that neglect might lead to an ulcer which could damage his sight (these cases are usually industrial ones and the hospital might be involved in compensation proceedings).

CARBOLIZATION OF CORNEAL ULCER

The surface of the corneal ulcer is touched with carbolic 80 per cent.

Requisites. Corneal loupe, speculum, watch glass, matchstick and

Investigations, Treatments and Minor Surgery

blotting paper. Drops of local anaesthetic, fluorescein and normal saline.

If the surgeon wishes to curette the surface of the ulcer before carbolizing, a small meibomian curette should be provided.

The eye must be thoroughly anaesthetised and then stained to show the exact area of ulceration.

After staining, the speculum should be put in and then the cornea must be dried with blotting paper. The tip of the sharpened matchstick should be dipped in carbolic, care being taken that it is not dripping; the whole area of the ulcer should be touched with carbolic, and it will turn white immediately. The blotting paper should be reapplied to prevent carbolic being spread over the eye by any flow of tears. It is usual to insert ointment or oily drops containing atropine before the speculum is removed and the lids are allowed to close. The procedure is not painful, but the patient may get some discomfort as the effect of the anaesthetic wears off. The matchstick is used because the soft wood absorbs just the right amount of carbolic: it should be sharpened to a blunt point. The cauterization of a dendritic corneal ulcer is often done with iodine instead of with carbolic, in which case, a drop of cocaine is allowed to fall on the area of iodized ulcer to neutralize any further effect of the treatment.

CAUTERIZATION BY METRICAUTERY

This treatment is occasionally used for corneal ulcers. The instrument is an electrical one and has a holder for a thermometer to register the temperature at the point of the instrument. After the use of local anaesthetic drops the point is applied to the cornea for one minute at a temperature of 75 to 90 deg C. The temperature is controlled by switching the current on and off, and it is convenient to heat it to 90 deg C and switch off before the application; the aim is to destroy organisms but not corneal tissue. The treatment is not painful nor is there usually subsequent discomfort.

INCISION AND CURETTAGE OF MEIBOMIAN CYST

A meibomian cyst, or chalazion, is a small painless lump near the lid margin. It is due to the blockage of the duct from the meibomian gland so that the secretion collects to form a small cyst. The cyst can

Investigations, Treatments and Minor Surgery

become inflamed and, if acutely so, it resembles a severe stye. Curettage is only performed if it is not inflamed.

Requisites.
Sterile Instruments:
Bard Parker knife, size No. 3 handle and 'E'-shape blade. See plate XXVIII.

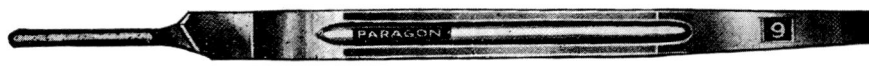

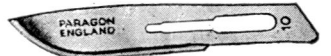

XXVIII. Scalpel handle with detachable blades

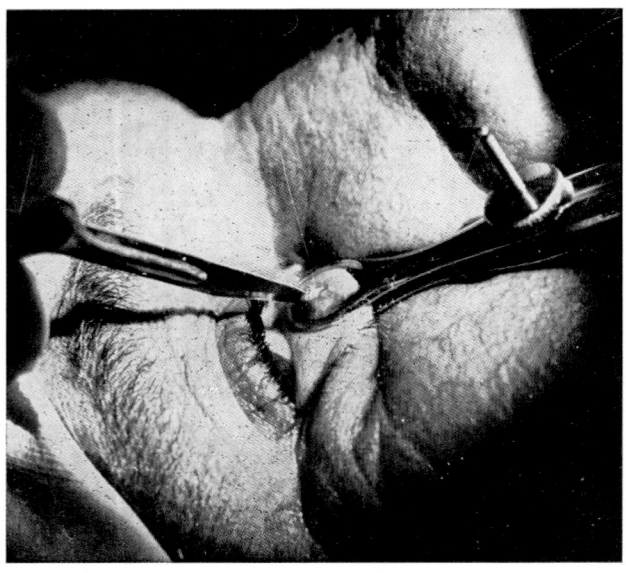

XXIX. Incision of meibomian cyst. The clamp is in position on the anaesthetized lower lid and the incision is through the conjunctival surface to be followed by curettage

Investigations, Treatments and Minor Surgery

  2 or 3 meibomian curettes of varying sizes
  Meibomian clamp.
Stitch scissors and conjunctival forceps may be required if there is fibrous tissue in the cyst wall to be excised.
  2 ml syringe, No. 17 needle and procaine with adrenaline for local injection.
  Local anaesthetic drops.
  Antiseptic to clean the skin.
  Sterile towel and swabs.

It is surprising how often young adults, especially men, feel faint during this minor operation, and if it can be conveniently arranged it is well to have the patient lying on a couch. He should be told that he will be given a small injection into the lid and that he will feel very little (see plate XXIX).

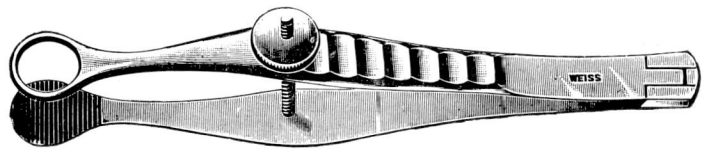

MEIBOMIAN CLAMP (Actual size)

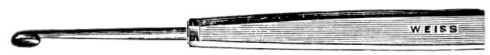

MEIBOMIAN CURETTE (Actual size)

The after treatment varies with the surgeon: it is always wise to give the patient a pad to hold on the eye immediately the operation is finished. If he presses on it for a few minutes any slight bleeding will be stopped and the eye can be swabbed quite clean before the patient goes home. If an irrigation is ordered, and the cyst was of the upper lid, the lid should be everted during the washout.

Opinion varies as to whether the eye should be covered for an hour or two, and, if so, as to whether to use an eyepad or a lint flap. It is undesirable for the eye to remain covered but patients may be

Investigations, Treatments and Minor Surgery

self-conscious at the bruised appearance of the lid and, if given a pad, they may keep the eye covered for several days.

It is usual for the patient to be kept under observation until all bleeding has stopped and then to have antibiotic ointment put in before leaving the hospital. Complications include corneal abrasion, if a pad was applied and the anaesthetized eye was rubbed or opened under the pad. An unusual complication is haemorrhage, reactionary or secondary, which should be treated with a pressure bandage and observation until it has been arrested.

SUBCONJUNCTIVAL INJECTIONS

Small amounts of fluid can be injected between the conjunctiva and the sclera. Examples of drugs introduced in this way are antibiotics, steroid preparations, and Mydricaine. Mydricaine contains atropine, procaine and adrenaline in a five minim dose, and as a subconjunctival injection it is used in iritis as the most effective mydriatic when other means of dilating the pupil have failed.

Method. The eye must be thoroughly anaesthetized, and if iritis is present the absorption of cocaine drops is helped by the addition of adrenaline 1 in 1,000.

The patient should be lying comfortably and a good light is necessary.

Requisites;

1 ml or 2 ml syringe.

No. 20 needle for injecting, and a second needle if the solution is to be withdrawn from a rubber-topped container.

Speculum and conjunctival forceps are requested by a few surgeons, but it is usual to inject without their use.

Swabs.

Local anaesthetic drops.

The drugs for injection.

When the eye is anaesthetized the site for the injection is selected and it is usually in the lower part of the eye for a first injection, but above or to one side if subsequent ones are required.

If the injection is below, the patient is asked to look above his head, and with the lower lid drawn down the needle is passed under the conjunctiva into the space between the conjunctiva

Investigations, Treatments and Minor Surgery

and sclera. The syringe is held so that the first finger can make the injection smoothly without any change of grip. The conjunctiva will swell up in a considerable bleb and there may be a little subconjunctival haemorrhage, so that it is wise to warn the patient, so that he is not alarmed if he looks in a mirror afterwards. The injection is not painful as a rule, but some of the drugs cause subsequent pain; the antibiotics are sometimes given in a solution of procaine to relieve this pain. Mydricaine causes pain when given in the acute phase of iritis. If local heat is ordered after an injection the patient must be specially warned to keep the eye closed owing to the recent local anaesthesia.

RETRO-BULBAR INJECTION

Drugs are sometimes given by retro (behind) bulbar (the eye) injection for their effect on the ciliary ganglion. This procedure is most often done in the theatre in preparation for intra-ocular operations, but it may also be required in a casualty department; in the latter case the most frequent occasions would be alcohol injection for a blind and painful eye, or procaine and Duvadilan as an emergency measure for sudden loss of sight due to spasm or occlusion of the central retinal artery. This treatment is always done by a doctor. The injection is made using a 2 ml or 5 ml syringe and a special retrobulbar needle which is 2 inches long and of very fine bore—No. 20. The site of the injection is either through the skin of the lid or through the conjunctiva. If the doctor's technique is not known it is necessary to prepare lotion for cleansing the skin and local anaesthetic drops. The patient should be lying on a couch with his head slightly raised. There is often a paues of a few minutes between injecting the procaine solution and following it with alcohol or other drug. The patient is not usually distressed by the treatment but complications which occasionally result from it are ptosis, drooping of the upper lid, or proptosis from a retrobulbar haemorrhage which displaces the eyeball forward; the ptosis usually recovers spontaneously, and the haemorrhage will become absorbed, but is alarming to the patient when it occurs.

Investigations, Treatments and Minor Surgery

TONOMETRY

The tension inside the eyeball, the intra-ocular tension, is variable, being usually between 15 and 25 mm of mercury. This tension can be estimated with a tonometer, but it is frequently judged by palpation of the eyeball with the fingers. Accurate judgment needs much experience and sensitive fingers: ophthalmic surgeons readily admit that it is a difficult test where the variation from the normal is slight. As a rule the tension of the second eye can be taken as normal and the other one be compared with it; in bilateral glaucoma this is not the case. The normal eye is felt first: the patient is asked to look down so that the tips of the index fingers can dimple the eyeball above the cornea, through the lid. The other fingers of both hands should be lightly rested on the patient's forehead to steady the hands. The fingers should be side by side and touching each other; one should be kept still, pressing on the eye while with the second an attempt is made to indent the globe; the impression conveyed to the stationary finger must be appreciated. As in other matters thorough experience of the normal allows the recognition of departure from it.

The normal intra-ocular tension has been described as feeling like 'a ripe plum'. Gradations are expressed as: Tension Normal (Tn), T full, T+1, T+2, T+3, the last being stony hard. Diminished tension occurs after a perforating wound, sometimes after a severe blow on the eye, and to a marked degree in a diseased, shrunk eye. Gradations are T, T–1, T–2, T–3, the last being a very soft eye. The difficulty of appreciating the tension is increased if the lid is oedematous or the eye unusually tender.

There are various types of tonometer but the Schiötz is the one in general use in this country.

There is one model without weights and a second one with a set of 7·5, 10, and 15 gram weights. The latter instrument is preferred by some surgeons as giving several readings for comparison but the disadvantage is that the cornea is subjected to repetitions of the test.

Method. The patient should be lying on a couch or bed with his head horizontal. There is sometimes a difficulty if a patient is dyspnoeic but it is usually possible to raise him a little and arrange the

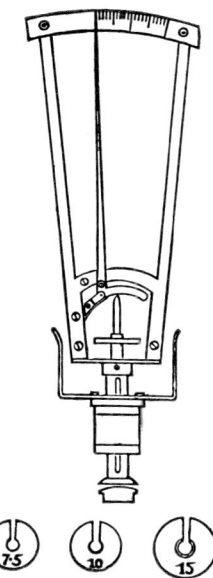

SCHIÖTZ TONOMETER WITH WEIGHTS

pillow so that his head is tilted back for the brief time the tonometry takes. Local anaesthetic drops must be those that do not alter the size of the pupil and for this reason cocaine is unsuitable. Decicaine or Holocaine are examples of suitable ones. A drop in each eye should be followed by a second drop in a minute or two and will usually suffice, but if the patient is hypersensitive it is better to use more drops and wait a few minutes.

The tonometer is balanced on the anaesthetized cornea and the stylet causes an indentation of the cornea; the depth of the indentation depends on the relative hardness of the eyeball so that the softer the eye the deeper the indentation. The stylet moves a pointer along a scale and the number which is shown on the scale can be translated by a graph to give a reading in millimetres of mercury. The eyelids should be controlled to hold the eye open without any pressure on the eye so that the tonometer rests on the centre of the cornea and the pointer should move evenly along the scale

Investigations, Treatments and Minor Surgery

until a steady reading is obtained. If the first reading shows an increase of tension or a marked change from previous ones the tonometry should be repeated to confirm the first result. If the doctor is easily available he may wish to check an unusual reading himself and it is usually appreciated if a nurse recognizes significant changes in tonometry readings and gives him the opportunity to repeat the test himself. Before use the tonometer should be held on the small testing disc to ensure that the pointer is moving freely and shows the zero reading. The testing disc has the same curvature as the corneal surface and as it is of metal it should give a reading of nought on the scale.

After use, the part of the tonometer which touched the eye should be cleaned by wiping it with a swab moistened with ether; ether is preferable to methylated spirit or Savlon because it evaporates so quickly. An alternative method of cleaning after use is to wipe the tonometer and then pass it through the flame of a spirit lamp. At intervals it will also be necessary to remove the stylet and clean it with ether and also clean the channel of the stylet by passing a pipe-cleaner soaked in ether up and down through it. The tonometers require very careful handling as the least bending of the lever will result in a false reading.

If a tonometer with weights is used it is necessary to have a pencil and rough paper at hand to jot down the different readings as they are made. It can be difficult to remember which reading was for the right eye and which for the left and it is a good habit to make a practice of always doing the right one first so that results are not muddled. It helps a patient to keep his eye still if he has something particular to look at with the eye which is not being tested. This can be a picture put on the ceiling or a finger held up by an assistant. If the patient's sight is poor it is quite satisfactory for him to be asked to hold his own hand above his face and look at his own finger.

Should a patient complain of acute pain about half an hour after the test it is possibly due to a corneal abrasion made by the tonometer and will require treatment and reassurance.

Aplanation Tonometer. This is another type of tonometer which is being increasingly used. The instrument measures the amount of pressure required to flatten a known area of cornea; and the harder

Investigations, Treatments and Minor Surgery

the eye the more pressure will be required. One type of aplanation tonometer is used attached to a slit lamp and another one can be used in the hand.

SCHIRMER'S TEST

This is a diagnostic test used in suspected Sjögren's disease which is characterized by symptoms of dry eyes and mouth. There is reduced secretion from the lacrimal glands and the test consists of inserting a strip of filter paper inside the lower lid and noting the distance on the strip which has become moistened in five minutes. If the production of tears is normal the moistening should be ten to fifteen millimetres from the lid margin, but in Sjögren's disease it may only be a few millimetres or nil. The strips of filter paper should be cut 50 millimetres in length and 5 millimetres in width and a bend should be creased 5 millimetres from one end; if the other end is marked with an R it will prevent a mistake over the right and left eyes when they are removed for measurement. The patient should be seated and the paper is then put inside the outer end of the lower lid of each eye and the patient asked to keep the eyes closed for five minutes. At the end of this time both papers are removed and the moistened part measured with a millimetre rule, deducting 5 millimetres for the part of the strip which was inside the closed lids.

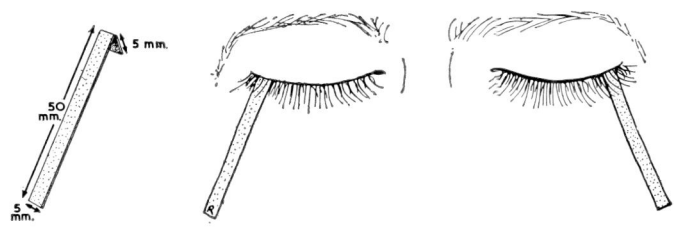

FILTER PAPER INSERTED FOR SCHIRMER'S TEST

CONTACT LENSES

Contact lenses resemble thin shells which fit the front surface of

Investigations, Treatments and Minor Surgery

the eye under the lids. The earlier contact lenses were made of glass but now they are nearly all of plastic material.

There are two indications for contact lenses. The first is visual and the second is therepeutic. The chief *visual indications* are extreme short sight, corneal irregularity such as conical cornea, and after cataract operation on one eye only. The advantage of a contact lens is that the lens is much closer to the eye than when it is in a spectacle frame which must clear the lids and the eye-lashes; if a lens is of high power, it alters the size of things seen and this discrepancy is reduced when the lens is very close to the eye. This fact is specially significant after an operation for cataract because the strong convex lens will magnify objects making it difficult to judge distances and, owing to the magnification, it is impossible to use an eye with normal sight in conjunction with one which has been operated on for cataract; the use of a contact lens will make the images sufficiently near the same size for both eyes to be used together again.

The *therapeutic indications* include corneal conditions such as mustard gas keratitis, insensitive corneae, corneal burns with adhesions of the lids to the eyeball and, sometimes, as a means of keeping a corneal graft in place in the immediate post-operative period. The contact lens may combine the functions of protecting the cornea and improving the sight of an eye.

There are two main types of contact lens in use at the present time, the haptic and the corneal lens (see plates XXX and XXXI).

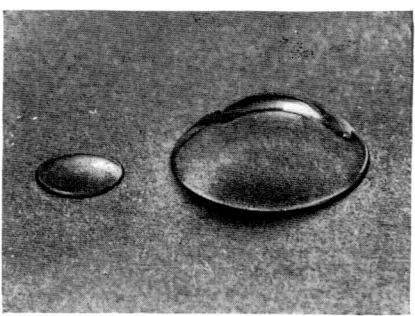

XXX. Corneal Lens and Haptic Lens: this photograph shows the comparative sizes of the lenses

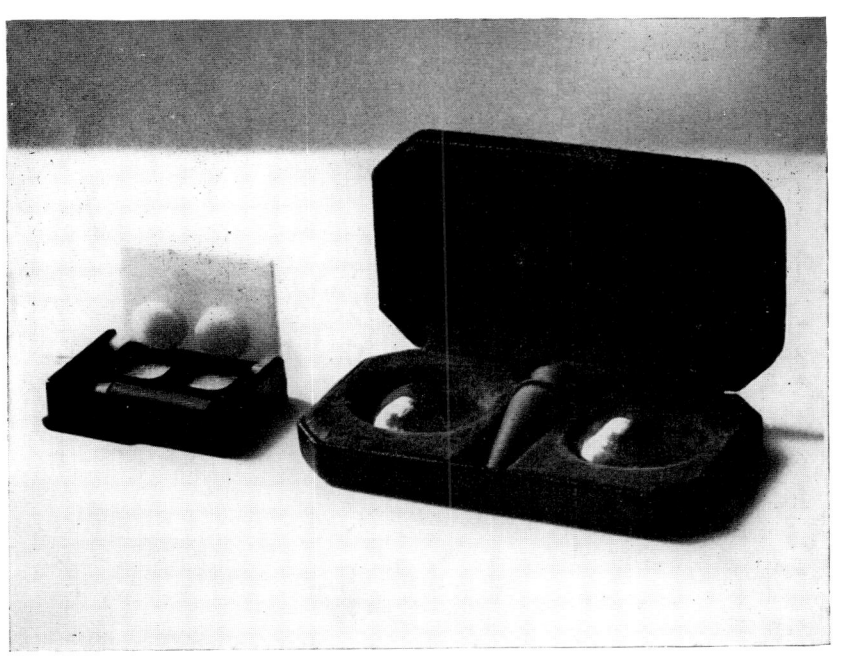

XXXI. Boxes of Contact Lenses and their suction holders

The Haptic Lens. This lens is the larger one in which the optical part is held in position over the cornea by a surround which rests on the 'white' of the eye. These lenses are sometimes made without a ventilating hole and they have to be worn with a solution filling the space between the lens and the cornea; this solution is similar in composition to tears. After a period of use, the sight may become misty and it is necessary to take the lens out and re-insert it with fresh solution. The alternative type of haptic lens is fenestrated and the tiny hole allows air and tears to pass through so that the cornea is ventilated.

The Corneal Lens. This is much smaller and it rests on the corneal surface; the lenses may be only eight millimetres in diameter. These lenses have the advantage of being completely invisible and they can usually be fitted more quickly but they are not suitable for all

XXXII. *Insertion of Haptic Contact Lenses*

The lens is held on the rubber suction holder of which the inside of the cup has been moistened and some of the air squeezed out. If the lens is not fenestrated, it will have been half filled with lotion. In the photograph the patient is now looking down and will approach the lens to the eye and slide the upper edge under the upper lid. She will then release the upper lid, draw down the lower lid, look upwards and at the same time will release the sucker by squeezing the bulb of the holder

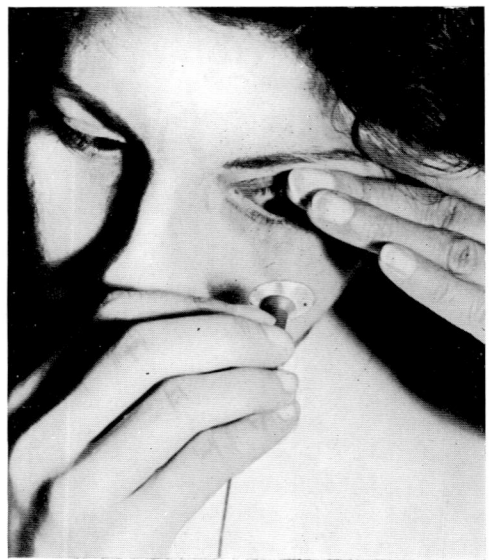

XXXIII. *The Removal of the Lens*

This photograph shows the lens just after it was lifted out of the eye. The method was to moisten the cup of the suction holder, squeeze all the air out and then press the holder gently on to the eye; when the pressure on the bulb was released it allowed the holder to be firmly attached to the lens. With a finger raising the upper lid and the eye looking down, the upper part of the lens was eased out of the eye as though hinged on the bottom edge

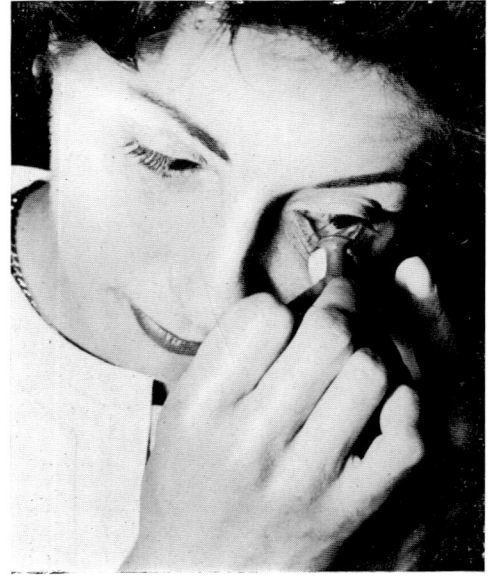

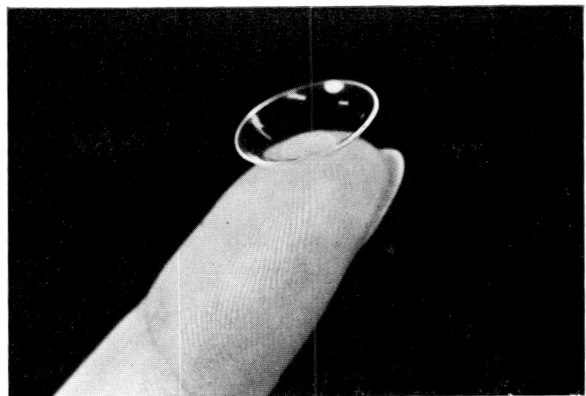

XXXIV. *Placing Corneal Contact Lens on the Eye*

Balance the cleaned and wetted lens on the right finger tip. Make sure that you place the lens with its concave side upwards

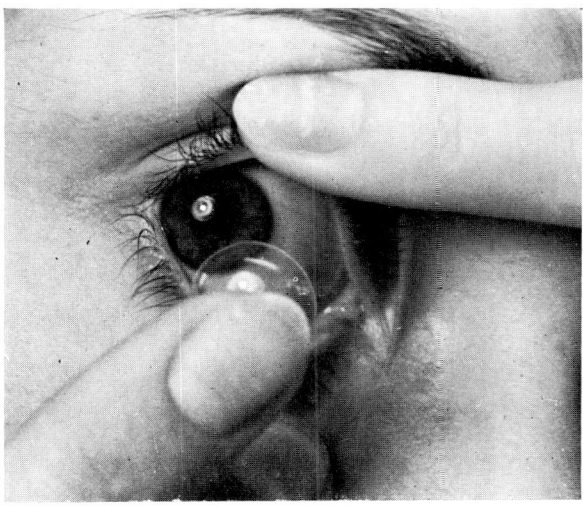

XXXV. *Placing Corneal Contact Lens on the Eye*

Separate the eyelids with the fingers of both hands in the way you find most convenient. Try to get as close to the lashes as possible

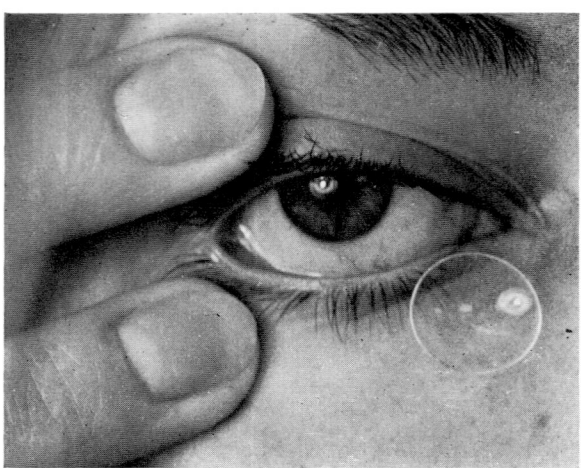

XXXVI. *Removal of the Corneal Contact Lens*
Separate the lids with two fingers and pull outwards, blinking as you do so; place the other hand below the chin to catch the lens

patients and are more easily lost (see plates XXXIV, XXXV and XXXVI).

Soft Contact Lens. This is slightly larger than the corneal lens and is made of a type of plastic capable of absorbing fluid and this property makes it flexible. The development is in its early stages at present; and the lens is not able to be used to correct astigmatism. It also requires very careful sterilization by boiling in a special container.

Contact lenses are not just an alternative to glasses for cosmetic reasons; they are very expensive owing to the expert fitting required for the individual person. The wearer has to overcome some initial discomfort and needs perseverance in the task of learning to handle them. The success depends largely on the skill with which the practitioner selects people he will accept as suitable patients; he will judge partly on the temperament and manual dexterity of the person but mostly on the motive for having them. The most successful wearers are those whose vision with ordinary glasses is very poor but is considerably improved with contact lenses; other successful wearers are

Investigations, Treatments and Minor Surgery

those whose career is dependent on not wearing glasses, for example, on the stage or in sport.

Under the British National Health Service, contact lenses may only be ordered for medical reasons on the recommendation of an ophthalmic consultant and the contact lens specialist will assess the suitability of the patient. They may be bought by private individuals but they are very expensive and the prospective buyer must bear in mind that considerable incentive and will power are necessary to wear them successfully and if these are not present, the money spent will be wasted. Contact lenses should never be bought or prescribed because of a passing idea.

A nurse is not qualified to give advice to a patient who is having difficulty in wearing contact lenses and he should be referred back to the practitioner who supplied them. However, patients sometimes attend a casualty department with acute pain in their eyes and they may be unable to remove the lenses. The pain is usually due to a corneal abrasion and the treatment consists of removing the lens, leaving it out, and treating the abrasion.

Method of Removing a Contact Lens (see plate XXXIII, p. 102)

A rubber suction holder is used to remove the lens, a larger size for the haptic lens and a smaller one for the corneal lens. The patient should be lying or sitting with the head resting back; he should be asked to look down while the upper lid is raised; the suction end of the holder is moistened and squeezed free of air and then applied to the surface of the contact lens towards twelve o'clock. With the patient keeping both eyes open and looking down, the lens is lifted downwards and out over the lower lid. If the eye is painful a few drops of local anaesthetic will be necessary before attempting the removal.

Care of Contact Lenses

The plastic material of which the lenses are made can be scratched if they are dried on coarse material and they can be bent out of shape if washed under too hot water; they can also be damaged by chemical solutions and for these reasons the practitioner who supplies the lenses will give careful instructions for the care and cleaning of them

Investigations, Treatments and Minor Surgery

and will also supply a special box in which the lenses and suction holder can be kept when not in use. A nurse may not receive these detailed instructions when dealing with a patient in an emergency but she will not damage the lenses if they are washed carefully in cold water, dried on a soft tissue and returned to the box. The lenses could be accidentally dropped down the waste of a wash basin if rinsed under a running tap.

If a patient is unable to wear the lenses for any reason, they may be left out but he may have to start wearing them for short periods until accustomed to them again.

Finally it can be stressed again that the people who wear contact lenses most successfully are those who obtain much better vision than when using glasses whereas those who choose them for cosmetic reasons often find that the discomfort is not worth the result.

5

BANDAGES AND SHADES

That a 'bad' eye should be covered by a pad and bandage is by no means a *sine qua non*.

The indications for covering an eye are:

1. *Corneal involvement:* this includes ulceration or injury, such as abrasion or foreign body. By keeping the lids closed over the eye, friction on the corneal surface is minimized and the epithelium is given the best opportunity to heal. Any corneal condition causes photophobia and this will also be relieved.

2. After most *operations* or *serious injuries* to the eye. The pad and bandage provide the needful protection and rest to the eye.

3. *After local anaesthesia,* opinion varies as to whether it is necessary to cover the eye. The arguments in favour of covering it are that normal blinking does not occur to keep the surface moist and, neither would a foreign body be felt. Against covering it, is the fact that the eye may not remain completely closed so that the pad can rub the insensitive cornea. Also, patients are inclined to keep the eye covered longer than necessary.

Contra-indications are:

1. *A discharging eye:* a covering pad would prevent the lids opening to allow discharge to escape and infection might be encouraged by keeping the eye warmer.

2. *An insensitive eye:* where corneal sensation is impaired the eye may open under the pad and the cornea could become rubbed.

It should be remembered that a pad and bandage prevents normal

Bandages and Shades

movement of the lids and the eye and is therefore undesirable unless necessary. The reduced field of vision and loss of stereoscopic vision are of considerable inconvenience. Most patients prefer not to have an eye covered.

There are various means of keeping a pad in place over the eye: a roller bandage, some type of special bandage, e.g. a Moorfield's Bandage, an eye shade or adhesive materials.

ROLLER BANDAGING

Roller bandaging for the eye presents several problems.

1. It is uncomfortable to have part of the head and hair covered.
2. If the patient is in bed the movement of the head on the pillow will disarrange a bandage unless it is covering a fairly large area and is firmly applied.
3. For a man employed in manual work, a white bandage becomes quickly soiled.
4. Patients object to such a conspicuous bandage.
5. A roller bandage is difficult for the patient to re-apply for himself.

Type of bandage. The gauze bandage is the cheapest and of little bulk.

The woven-edged variety is very satisfactory and is economical if the bandages are washed for repeated use.

The crepe bandage is the most comfortable, but too expensive for general use.

Width of bandage. $1\frac{1}{2}$ inch is the size most commonly used: if a 2 inch is preferred it is applied with fewer turns round the head.

SINGLE EYE BANDAGE (see plates XXXVII to XLI)

Securing the end of the bandage.

1. The end can be tucked under the last turn.
2. A safety pin can be used, but it must be put in the centre of the forehead. Safety pins should not be used for children.
3. Nurses like to use a small piece of adhesive strapping; this is

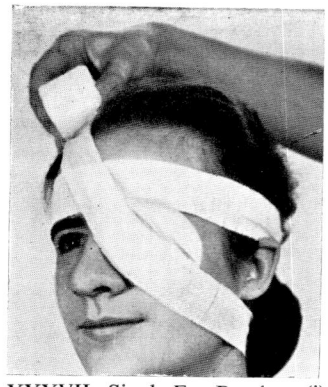

XXXVII. Single Eye Bandage (i)

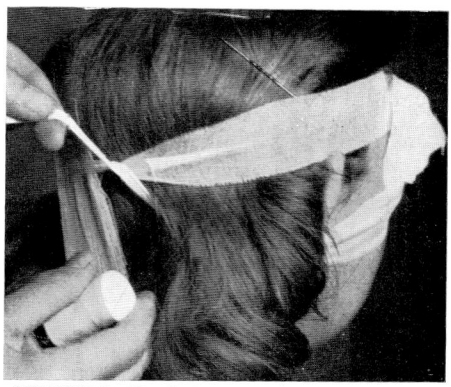

XXXVIII. Single Eye Bandage: alternative method (i)

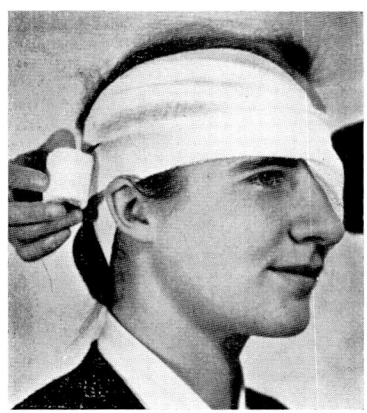

XXXIX. Single Eye Bandage (ii)

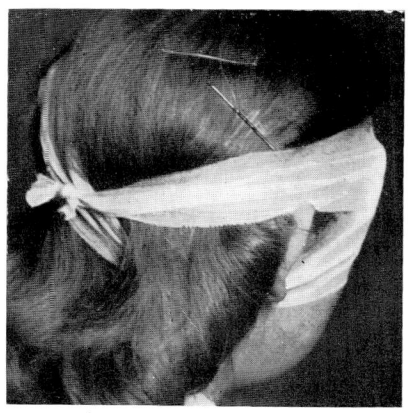

XL. Single Eye Bandage: alternative method (ii)

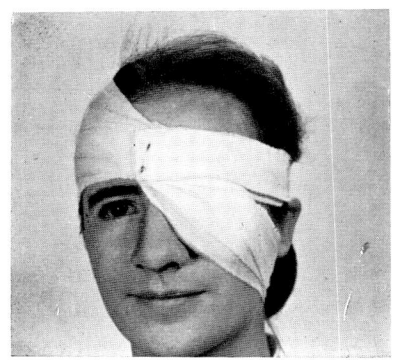

XLI. Single Eye Bandage (iii)

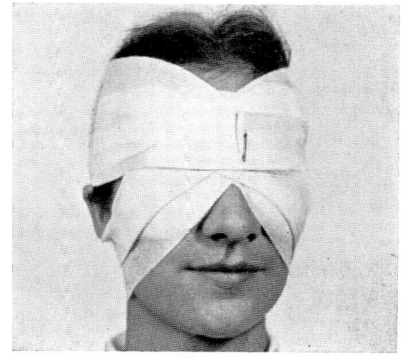

XLII. Double Eye Bandage

Bandages and Shades

neat and secure, but the adhesive material is tiresome to wash off the bandages.

Special points

1. The turns round the head must be taken below the occiput at the back to prevent the bandage rising off the head.

2. The turns should be carefully under the lobe of the ear and not dragging it out of place or covering the ear.

3. The turns round the forehead should be well above the eyebrows so that there is no chance of interfering with the second eye.

4. A minimum length of bandage should be applied. Where woven edged bandages are used it is convenient to keep a small stock of shorter ones.

SINGLE EYE BANDAGE, ALTERNATIVE METHOD

See plates XXXVIII and XL.

This method of application is very useful in out-patient work for cases which require a bandage that need not be re-applied at home, for example, for an eye from which the pad and bandage can be discarded in a few hours or one which is seen daily and requires no treatment at home.

The advantages are that it can be applied very securely even with a cheap gauze bandage, and it is of minimum bulk under a hat.

DOUBLE EYE BANDAGE (see plate XLII)

This is not often used owing to the greater comfort and convenience of the Moorfield's Bandage.

TYPES OF SPECIAL BANDAGES FOR SINGLE EYE

1. *Knitted Bandage* (see plate XLIII).

Knitting Pattern. No. 8 Knitting Cotton and No. 13 needles. Cast on 8 stitches. Knit plain for 8 rows.

9th row. Knit 2, increase once, knit to last 3 stitches, increase once, knit 2.

12th, 15th, 18th, 21st, 24th and 27th rows like 9th, others plain (22 stitches).

8 rows plain.

35th row. Knit 2, knit 2 together, knit to last 4 stitches, knit 2 together, knit 2.

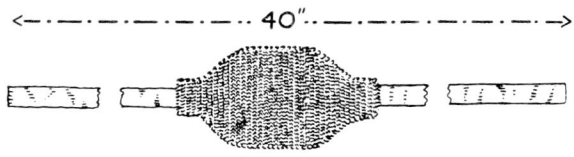

Knitted Bandage

38th, 41st, 44th, 50th and 53rd, like 35th (8 stitches), others plain.
Knit 8 rows plain.
Cast off.

There are many other patterns of knitted bandages and on the whole the wider the tape or knitted strip, the better the bandage will stay in position. At present there is no machine-made article and they must be made by hand.

This type of bandage is widely used and can easily be applied by the patient. It is washable and allows ventilation to the eye pad. On some patients, probably owing to the shape of the head, the tape tends to slip down over the other eye in an uncomfortable manner. For a woman a Kirbigrip will help to keep it in position, but for those patients on whom it does not remain in place it is better not to persevere with its use.

There is a need for the invention of a good type of single eye bandage which will keep a pad securely in position, is easy for the patient to apply, is washable and cheap.

SPECIAL TYPES FOR BOTH EYES

Moorfield's Bandage. For dressing the eyes the side tapes are drawn forwards and the bandage turned up on the forehead. In this way the head need not be raised from the pillow. See plate XLIV.

The Moorfield's Bandage is ideal for its purpose and is very widely used.

Many-tail of 2 inch Crepe Bandage. This bandage gives a firmer pressure over the pads. It can be used for children after operation for squint.

EYE SHADES

Black Eye Shade. There is a well-known pattern of black shade

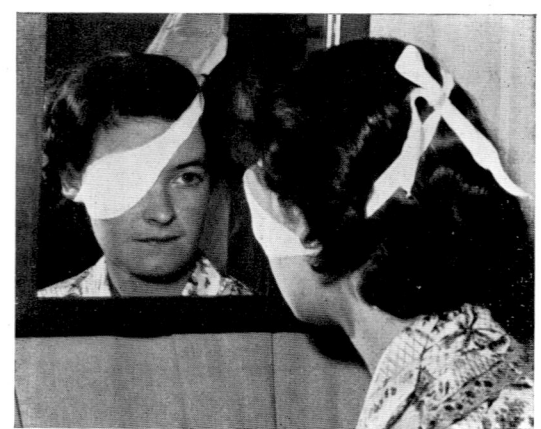

XLIII. Knitted Eye Bandage

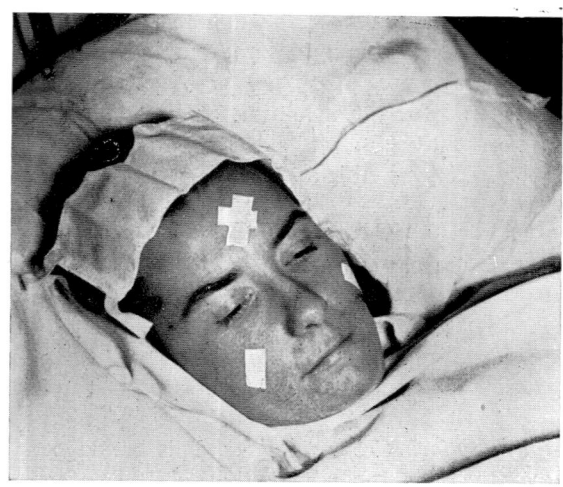

XLIV. Moorfield's Double Eye Bandage: turned up while the eyes are dressed

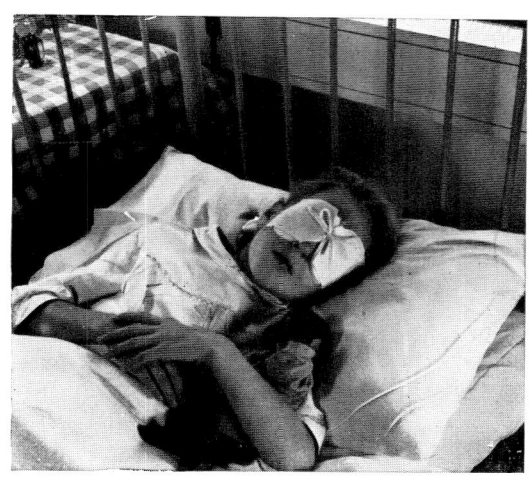

XLV. Double Eye Elastoplast 'Gate' Dressing

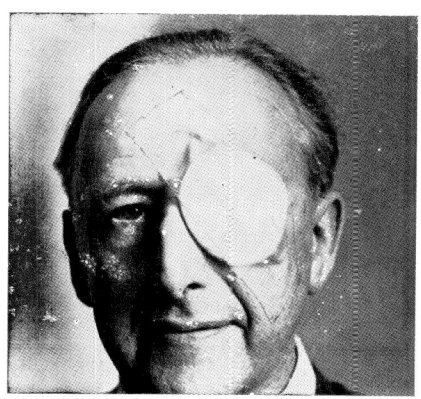

XLVI. An adhesive material, Blenderm used as an alternative to a bandage

H

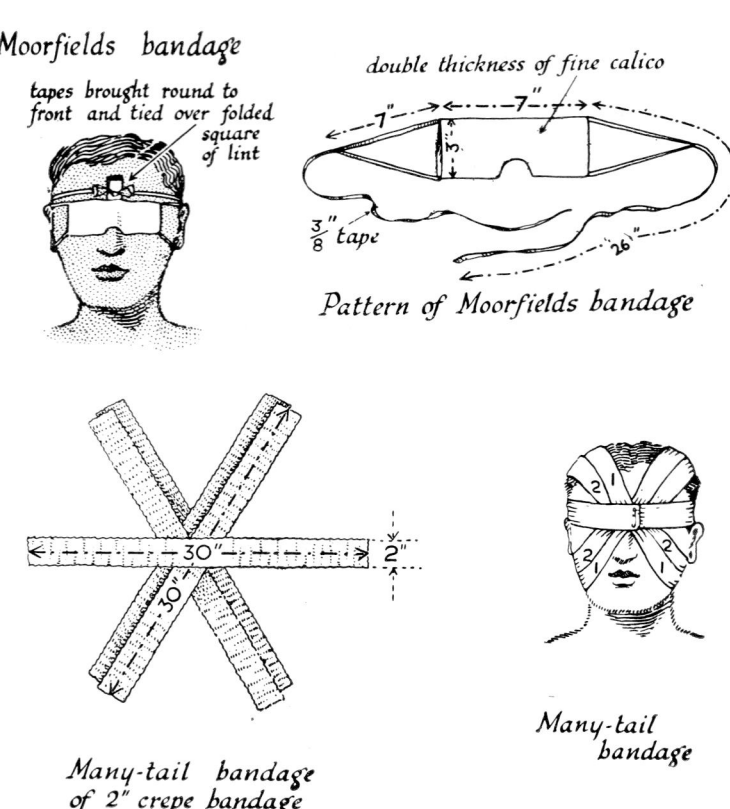

Moorfields bandage

tapes brought round to front and tied over folded square of lint

double thickness of fine calico

Pattern of Moorfields bandage

Many-tail bandage of 2" crepe bandage

Many-tail bandage

lined with green silk material. The shade is comfortable to wear and does not show the dirt. The serious disadvantage is that it is relatively expensive and the patient is unlikely to discard such a valuable article when it becomes slightly soiled with discharge; for this reason it is looked upon with disfavour by hospital staffs.

Pink Celluloid Shade. These are cheap and washable and well liked by men doing manual work. Their disadvantage is that they do not allow ventilation to the eye pad; if the eye is watering the warm damp pad will remain in contact with the lids. Many ophthalmic departments forbid their use for this reason, but they have a value for

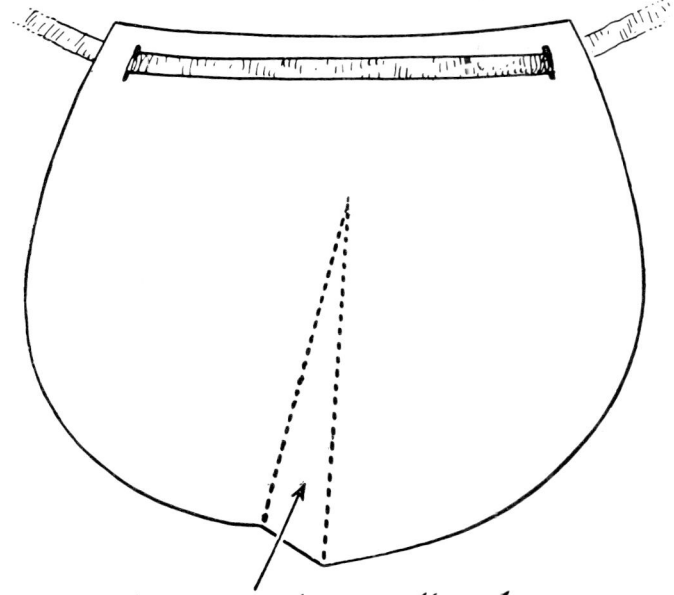

Pattern (full size) of Cardboard Shade

pleat stitched in cardboard

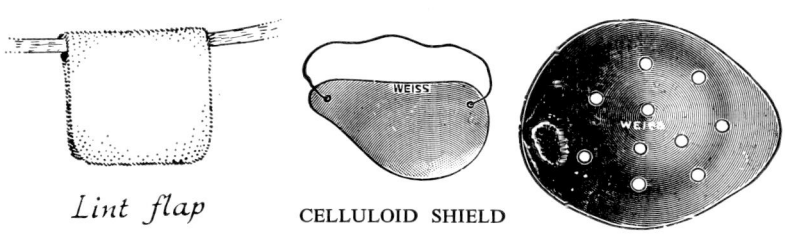

Lint flap   CELLULOID SHIELD   CARTELLA SHIELD

Bandages and Shades

covering the eye when a pad is not necessary, for example, in the relief of diplopia or the covering of a socket.

Cardboard Shades. These can be made of thin white cardboard, threaded with tape or fine elastic. They are serviceable and cheap.

Cartella Shield. These are made for the right and left eyes. They are of plastic material and are kept in position with adhesive strapping. They are useful for covering an insensitive eye and are sometimes put over the eye pad for additional protection after cataract operation.

Lint Flap. A double fold of lint can be kept in place by bandage tied round the head or by adhesive strapping to the forehead. They are very useful if pressure on the eye is to be avoided, but are apt to become untidy, especially if worn out-of-doors.

Adhesive Materials. Eye pads can be kept in place by strips of adhesive material. These have the advantage of holding the pad securely in place without pressure on the eye. For inspection of the eye the strapping should be cut at the top of the pad and a short length can be reapplied over the previous piece; in the same way a fresh pad can be put on by putting new strapping over that already on the skin. The adhesive materials are difficult to secure to a man's cheek unless he is shaved regularly and they occasionally cause a local skin irritation. 'Gate' dressings of Elastoplast can be used over single or double pads and are very useful for a child (see plate XLV).

The ideal adhesive strapping should be firm enough to give support, not irritant to the skin, be available in convenient widths, and not too expensive. It is an advantage if the roll can be held in some type of dispenser so that lengths can be torn off leaving the end free to pick up. Any adhesive which remains on the skin must be easy to remove (see plate XLVI).

Dark Glasses. Dark Glasses are frequently used in the treatment of eye diseases. Crookes lenses are scientifically tinted to cut out particular parts of the light spectrum; they are of different colours denoted by letters and of different darkness denoted by numbers, for example, Crookes B2 is smoke-coloured and the one often used for sun glasses. Polaroid glasses break up the rays of light and thus reduce their dazzling effect. There are various designs of clip-on dark

Bandages and Shades

glasses which can be worn over ordinary spectacles and the most comfortable are the lightest in weight. It is sometimes asked whether dark glasses need to be the expensive ones; the very cheap ones sometimes have flaws in the glass which might cause distortion and also the tinting may be dark but not effective in absorbing the ultra-violet light rays.

Dark glasses are often ordered for the relief of photophobia after operations on the eyes and patients who are being treated with drops which dilate the pupil will need protection from bright light. They have cosmetic uses when patients are sensitive about the appearance of an eye, for example, when the lids are treated with gentian violet. The wearing of dark glasses can become a habit so that normal eyes feel the need of them unnecessarily. People who are very fair will require them more than those with darker colouring.

Green Tennis Shades are sometimes valuable as a means of protection against light; this might be the case if dark glasses could not be worn because of a skin condition or a rodent ulcer near the nose, or because the shape of the face makes spectacles uncomfortable.

The shading provided by the brim of a hat or a sports shade is particularly desirable for those who have early cataract; the patient realizes that he sees better when his eyes are shaded from bright light, and he will often put on dark glasses. It should be explained to him that a bright light on his eyes will affect his sight. A useful simile is that of a dirty windscreen which will obscure the driver's vision slightly in ordinary light, but will be much worse when the sun is shining directly on it; the slight opacity in the lens of his eye will have the same effect and he will be helped more by shading the eyes than by wearing dark glasses.

6

NOTES ON CASUALTY AND OUT-PATIENT WORK

NOTES ON CASUALTY WORK

A lot of accidents involve the face and eyes and a number of eye conditions occur suddenly or become worrying at short notice, so that there is a considerable volume of work which must be dealt with under casualty conditions. In addition to the ophthalmic hospitals every general hospital and general practitioner attends to these casualties, and district nurses and occupational health nurses have to advise and treat them. The following are the most usual conditions for which patients seek casualty treatment.

Variety of Emergencies

Emergencies fall into three main groups:

(1) an accident involving the eye;
(2) acute pain;
(3) sudden loss of vision.

ACCIDENTS

Accidents may be trivial or serious but the patient is usually terrified of losing his sight, especially if both eyes are involved. One of the first casualty duties is to record the vision of each eye separately; besides its medical value, this often reassures the patient. Many accidents result in compensation claims and the vision recorded at the first attendance is very important.

Notes on Casualty and Out-patient Work

Foreign Bodies

Foreign bodies are one of the most common causes of injury.

Subtarsal Foreign Body

A piece of grit under the upper lid is very painful as it scratches the cornea each time the eye moves. The eversion of an upper lid and removal of the foreign body is valuable first aid. In hospital there are the advantages of a good light and magnifying equipment. A damp swab stick is used to wipe away the foreign body and a special stain, fluorescein, is used to show if there has been any corneal injury; if this has occurred the treatment would include a firm pad and bandage which assists healing and relieves pain.

Corneal Foreign Body

Tiny particles sometimes become stuck to the surface of the cornea; if not removed they cause an inflammation of the eye and also leave a permanent scar and if the scar is over the pupil it may affect the sight of the eye. A corneal foreign body is removed with a sharp pointed instrument after local anaesthesia with drops such as amethocaine, and the patient is seen regularly until healing is complete.

Intra-ocular Foreign Body

Occasionally a foreign body perforates the cornea or sclera and remains inside the eye (see page 216). This is a very serious injury although not necessarily a painful one. The patient will require X-ray, admission to hospital and operation.

Corneal Abrasions

Corneal abrasions are caused in various ways, such as a wire springing back and hitting the eye, or a baby's finger-nail scratching the mother's eye. The transparency of the cornea is essential to sight, and the extreme pain these abrasions cause is a valuable protective mechanism because it makes the patient seek treatment. The treatment will include an ointment to act as an antiseptic and lubricant and a firm pad and bandage.

Accidents in which a person is buried or showered with dust or sand may result in the surface of the eyes being covered with the small particles. They have usually caused corneal damage so that the eyes are very painful and water profusely. After local anaesthetic drops, the eyes are irrigated thoroughly and the lids everted and washed to remove all the foreign bodies. It may take some time to carry out this treatment but as a rule there are no serious after-effects.

Blows on the Eye

A 'black eye' is bruising of the lids and surrounding tissues; it may cause alarm but the orbital bones often take the force of the blow and may be fractured. The lids may be too swollen for the eye to open but, if the lid is gently raised, the vision test is a useful indication as to whether the eye has been damaged. A blow sometimes causes *haemorrhage inside the eye* and this must be treated with respect as it is difficult to tell how much damage has been done until the blood has cleared. Rest in bed, at home or in hospital, is necessary.

Perforating Injury

A blow on the eye which cuts through the cornea or sclera is a *perforating injury*: accidents with bows and arrows, shotguns or scissors are common causes. It is always very serious and requires immediate admission and operation; sight after such an injury is seldom very good.

Lacerations of the Eyelids

Lacerations of the eyelids need expert suturing to prevent scars which cause irregularity of the lid margin so that lashes turn inwards and irritate the eye; if the cut is in the inner corner of the lids the tear passages may have been involved.

Burns

Burns are often much worse than they appear at first and the chemical ones such as ammonia or lime burns, are specially serious. The permanent damage to be feared is that due to corneal scars and lid deformities. If the injury is caused by lime or a splash of corrosive fluid into the eye, the nurse's first duty on receiving the patient is to wash the face and eyelids thoroughly with water and then to put in a few drops of local anaesthetic and irrigate very thoroughly with normal saline. Ophthalmological opinion nowadays stresses the value of very thorough washing rather than reliance on chemical antidotes. The patient is often suffering from shock and, if the skin of the face is involved, specially gentle handling is needed in order to inspect and treat the eyes; this is more easily done if the patient is lying down and the doctor usually puts in anaesthetic drops before examination. If both eyes are involved the patient is usually admitted for at least 24 hours.

Flash Burns or Welder's 'Arc Eye'

Flash burns from ultra-violet light cause superficial corneal damage with a delay in the onset of pain for several hours after exposure. The watering and pain makes it difficult to open the eyes and patients often come in certain that they have been blinded. The injury is seldom very serious and local anaesthetic drops and reassurance will relieve the immediate distress. The condition usually clears up within 24 hours but the precaution of wearing protective goggles when exposed to ultra-violet light should be stressed.

Firework Injuries

The damage caused by fireworks may be a combination of burns, foreign bodies, corneal abrasions and possibly a perforating wound; the patients are often children and both eyes may be involved.

ACUTE PAIN IN THE EYE

Acute pain brings patients into a casualty department but, apart from accidents, there are not many common causes.

Acute Glaucoma

Acute glaucoma is probably the commonest cause of sudden onset of very severe pain. Glaucoma is the condition of raised pressure in the eyeball; it may develop gradually without symptoms and the patient is often first aware of it when he has an acute attack. As well as the pain, he feels ill and nauseated and it is typical that he feels so bad that he does not mind what happens to him in the way of admission and operation. This is an emergency: correct diagnosis and prompt treatment to control the pressure may prevent permanent

Notes on Casualty and Out-patient Work

loss of sight. The treatment will include frequent instillation of miotic drops, such as eserine and systemic Diamox although this frequently increases the nausea before relieving the pain. Admission is often required but if an operation is suggested the nurse must be careful not to assure the relatives that it will completely cure the glaucoma as the eye may already have been damaged.

Other conditions which cause acute pain are *acute iritis*, *corneal ulcers*, *shingles* of the forehead and *acute infection* of the lids.

Patients often come to an eye hospital with severe pain 'in the eye' and are found to have acute frontal sinusitis.

SUDDEN LOSS OF SIGHT

When patients come in with sudden loss of sight in one eye the most common causes are retinal detachment and retinal haemorrhage or thrombosis. These conditions require urgent treatment although it may not be possible to restore the sight.

Retinal detachment occurs most often in short-sighted people. The treatment is admission for operation.

Retinal vessel thrombosis is associated with hypertension and is a medical problem, the eye condition being dependent on the general health. Similarly *retinal haemorrhages* occur frequently in diabetic patients, and the treatment of the eye is that of the disease.

Rupture of the optic nerve may be caused by a fractured base of skull and inevitably results in complete and permanent loss of sight in an otherwise perfect eye; this is one of the most tragic accidents.

OTHER PROBLEMS

Diplopia (double vision), if of sudden onset, is an emergency as it may be caused by pressure from behind, displacing the eye; the cause could be a rapidly growing cerebral tumour or a serious infection of the orbit and either would require immediate attention.

Patients also come to a casualty department with problems like the inability to remove their contact lenses, and they may be in pain from corneal abrasions.

The loss of glasses is a desperate plight to a very short-sighted person as he cannot see to get about or even to look for them. As a

Notes on Casualty and Out-patient Work

temporary measure, he can prick a hole in a card and hold it close to his eye and he can then see quite well.

In addition to the above there are many minor eye diseases which have an acute onset and are often treated in hospital casualty departments. These include acute conjunctivitis, acute iritis, corneal ulcers, cysts of lids and allergies. The treatment required gives scope for nursing skill including advising patients how to carry out the instructions they are given, and it provides most satisfying work combined with excellent opportunities for teaching nurses.

CASUALTY EQUIPMENT

The equipment of a casualty department will depend on the size of the department and on the volume of work. If the eye conditions are seen in a general accident department the minimum requirements are a couch and an inspection lamp on a stand or bracket similar to an Anglepoise lamp. A test type of letters properly illuminated is necessary (see pages 22 and 24 for the distance required). There must be some type of magnifying loupe and an ophthalmoscope.

INSTRUMENTS

For examinations and treatments a selection of the instruments listed would be required (see p. 209).

DRUGS

The special drugs required will be mostly in the form of drops and ointments, and naturally the variety and quantity will depend on the work undertaken.

At a minimum *Eye Drops* should include the following:

For anaesthesia—Cocaine 4 per cent and Decicain 1 per cent or another drug which does not dilate the pupil in the way cocaine does.

For dilating the pupil—homatropine 2 per cent, and atropine 1 per cent.

For contracting the pupil—pilocarpine 1 per cent, and eserine 1 per cent.

For haemostasis—adrenaline 1 in 1,000.

Notes on Casualty and Out-patient Work

Antibiotic drops such as Albucid 10 per cent, penicillin 25,000 units/ml, or other drugs.

Normal saline drops are useful for washing out fluorescein stain.

Eye ointments, should include an antibiotic one such as Albucid 10 per cent, or Neomycin ½ per cent, and a steroid one such as Betnesol.

Other requirements will be Fluorescein staining solution or impregnated papers, and an anaesthetic solution for local injection, such as Lignocaine 2 per cent, with adrenaline 1 in 10,000.

DRESSINGS

These should include eye pads, swabs, prepared swab sticks, 1½-in. or 2-in. gauze bandages, and adhesive materials.

Other equipment would be an undine, one pint measure jug, small kidney receiver, and a protective cape for irrigations.

For an industrial surgery a selection of the above equipment would be made according to the work undertaken.

The casualty department of an ophthalmic hospital would be more elaborately equipped. In addition to treatment couches some hospitals favour dental chairs for carrying out minor procedures. Treatment chairs should have adjustable head rests and modified operating lamps must be provided. If possible there should be a small rest or recovery room where patients can sit in comfort under observation.

NOTES ON OUTPATIENT WORK

Out-patient departments vary very much in the pattern of their organization and therefore in the responsibilities and duties of the nursing staff. At present a sister is usually in charge of the organization of clinics and this includes getting the patients in to see the doctors, and seeing that the medical notes are complete with recent reports and X-rays, etc. She is also responsible for the care of all equipment and the ordering of repairs and replacements, and for seeing that the premises are cleaned and kept in good order. It may well be that in the future all the above work may be the responsibility of someone who is not a trained nurse; the work might be

Notes on Casualty and Out-patient Work

done with better continuity because nursing staff are frequently moved from one department to another for their own experience or for relief purposes, and female nurses are seldom good with complicated electrical equipment. The advantage of nurses being in charge is in their contact with the patients and the doctors, and the work provides very good opportunities for keeping knowledge up to date and for teaching. Trained nurses may be in a position to advise about planning or reorganizing departments and experience previously gained makes it much easier to visualize future requirements. If the nursing staff is in charge of the equipment the sister must acquaint herself with the use of each instrument; most of these are electrical and it is necessary to know the correct voltage or battery required. It is usual to have transformers to reduce the voltage from the mains electricity to 3, 6, or 12 volts according to the requirements of the instrument. There are so many different bulbs to be kept in stock that the sister needs to check the reserves carefully and work in close co-operation with the hospital electrician. When preparing for clinics it is advisable to switch on every piece of apparatus to test it and so allow time for necessary repairs before work starts. The quantity of flexes and connections makes the routine cleaning and dusting very difficult unless every instrument is unplugged and either put away or covered up after each clinic.

It is usual for doctors to have some drop bottles on their desks so that they can put in mydriatic drops or stain an eye with fluorescein, but the sister will also need a duplicate stock. There must be a room with a couch or an adjacent treatment room and a darkened cubicle. There is sometimes a minor operation theatre run in conjunction with the out-patient department.

In an ophthalmic hospital certain arrangements depend on whether medical teaching is undertaken. An appointment system is necessary but difficult to organize successfully as many patients may require a number of different tests and examinations during one attendance, and the surgeon will have to see the various results before completing his examination. The staff working in connection with the clinic will include orthoptists, refracting and dispensing opticians in addition to nurses, medical social worker, pharmacist and reception clerks, and good overall supervision is required to prevent patients waiting

Notes on Casualty and Out-patient Work

longer than necessary. Most patients would prefer to have all the tests at one attendance if possible but the inconvenience is worse if one is not expecting a prolonged visit.

There are often several doctors working at once and they may be in separate rooms or in one large room divided into cubicles and sharing equipment such as slit-lamps, perimeters and Bjerrum screens. It might appear better for doctors to work alone but there is a certain advantage in their being able to consult each other easily. In hospital practice the consultants must be assisted by younger men who are gaining their experience, and in these circumstances a consultant is helped to keep in touch with patients he is unable to see himself, if he is shown all the medical notes at the start of the session.

Whether the organization of the clinic is in the hands of nursing staff or not, there is much nursing work connected with it. A sister will be responsible for carrying out or supervising many of the tests and treatments. These would include tonometry readings, syringing of lacrimal sacs, Schirmer's tests, epilation of lashes, instillation of drops and observation of the results, and a variety of other work. There will also be medical tests such as urinalysis, recording of blood-pressures, etc. Most surgeons welcome a sister's co-operation in observing significant facts and asking his advice if treatments are not straightforward to carry out, or tests produce unusual results. There is scope for utilizing nursing skill and experience and excellent opportunities to learn more of eye diseases and their investigations. Hospitals vary very much in what work is considered to be within the province of an ophthalmic-trained nurse; sometimes minor operations such as incision and curettage of meibomian cysts, opening a tarsorrhaphy, or electrolysis of lashes, are entrusted to a sister and sometimes a casualty sister sees and treats a patient who has a foreign body in the eye. In some hospitals peripheral field tests are delegated to nurses. Very much depends on the experience of the nursing staff, on the availability of doctors and on the numbers of patients to be dealt with.

The eye clinic in a general hospital would be organized very differently. It would probably be held only once or twice a week in a consulting room which served other purposes. The doctor would

Notes on Casualty and Out-patient Work

probably be a consultant working on his own and the sister would not necessarily have had special ophthalmic training. In these circumstances the nursing staff would help as much as possible by preparing patients for tests and treatments to be carried out by the doctor. The patients benefit by receiving expert opinion and being seen by the same doctor at each visit, but it is extravagant of a consultant's time and he is handicapped by lack of assistants and equipment. It would be important that the nurse in charge of such a clinic should be allowed to continue the work as the doctor would rely on her. This clinic would be good for student nurses to observe with the help of a clinical instructor who had ophthalmic experience.

PART II

7

NURSING OF IN-PATIENTS

In *General Hospitals* the number of ophthalmic patients is comparatively small and as it will include men, women and children they are often in different parts of the hospital. It is ideal if a small unit can be used for eye work and the best use can be made of it if the partitioning allows the use of beds for men or women as the changing circumstances require.

In Ophthalmic Hospitals it would seem that 'progressive care' wards would be of benefit by allowing the first few pre- and postoperative days to be spent in wards under the care of trained nurses for the twenty-four-hour span, while the subsequent days would be better catered for if spent in a unit which included day rooms and a dining-room shared by men and women with a relatively simple type of sleeping accommodation. The ward unit should be on the same floor as the operating theatre, and the second stage unit could conveniently be near the kitchen. It must be borne in mind that most of the in-patients are old and many need help with washing and dressing and going to the toilet, but this care can be given by suitable nursing assistants supervised by trained nurses.

Ward Requirements

The ward and day rooms must be warm enough for old people to sit in comfort. Lighting should be arranged so that no patient lies looking into a light; it is ideal to have individual lights over each bed and a system of concealed general lighting which is sufficiently bright to prevent a dim, depressing effect. Electric points over each

Nursing of In-Patients

bed allow equipment such as examination lights or Maddox heaters to be used.

Polished floors are particularly dangerous for old people and are noisy or squeaky at night. An easily washable flooring like Vinyl tiles is good.

Blinds or curtains should be effective in keeping out sunlight if necessary and also in allowing examination of patients in a dim light.

If *beds* are of the usual height for hospital use there must be sets of steps to allow old people to climb in and out. In a unit for second stage post-operative patients the beds could be of the height in use at home. If there are a few beds of adjustable height they will be useful for the more helpless and the elderly arthritic patients.

Bedside lockers should be of a design which does not require stooping or kneeling to reach the contents. Clothing accommodation should allow every patient to keep his indoor clothes in the ward unit.

Bedside tables which swing across the bed are convenient for meals in bed.

Washing Facilities. In addition to bathrooms there should be curtained cubicles where patients could sit at a low wash basin. The cubicles should have enough space for a helper with the patient if necessary and a low-level sink for washing legs and feet. The modern type of bathing chair with spray attachments would be useful (see plate XLVII). Whatever accommodation is provided it must be remembered that old people are slow and there must be a generous proportion of washing-cubicles.

Lavatories should be large enough to allow a helper to take a patient in and should have handles to allow patients to help themselves off the lavatory seat. The practice of allowing old people to go to the lavatory makes it more likely that some may feel unwell or collapse when in there, and there should be arrangements whereby the door can be opened outwards or an upper half be opened like a stable door because it is impossible to get into a small lavatory if the patient has fallen forwards and the door opens inwards.

A Treatment Room attached to the ward is ideal; many patients can go to it for routine treatments. If it is fitted with a special treatment chair and an Anglepoise lamp, it allows work to be done under

Cataract Nursing

to part with a tight vest or combinations which would add considerably to nursing difficulties later on. It is much more convenient for extra clothing to be added over the gown.

Women's long hair is best arranged in two plaits. Opportunity should be taken to wash it before operation as this will be inadvisable for a few weeks afterwards.

Men should be warned not to shave themselves for several days after the operation.

The local preparation for the eye used to include a saline irrigation but this is not usual now owing to the use of antibiotic drops at frequent intervals. The lids and surrounding area should be cleaned with a cleansing lotion such as Savlon, and mydriatic drops will depend on the individual surgeon's preferences, as it may be required to have the pupil fully dilated or only half dilated. A lint flap is sometimes put over the eye following the skin preparation. Local anaesthetic drops will be ordered to be instilled at a few-minute intervals twenty minutes before operation unless a general anaesthetic is given; cocaine 4 per cent and adrenaline 1 in 1,000 is usual and it is important that the eye is kept closed because cocaine will cause a drying of the cornea if the eye is open.

POST-OPERATIVE NURSING

The aim is to allow the section to heal without the edges becoming separated; this usually takes place in about five days, but would be delayed by extreme old age, intercurrent disease, e.g. diabetes.

To this end the following must be avoided:

Restlessness is best prevented by constant attention to the patient's needs and desires; for this reason the allocation of staff to these wards must be adequate.

Squeezing the eye. This might be due to sudden noise or movement, as from a door slamming or the bed being jarred.

A patient is inclined to squeeze his eye during the dressing of it if the lid is held roughly or a drop falls without warning.

Straining occurs during coughing, vomiting, or in an endeavour to pass a constipated stool. For nausea an intramuscular injection of Fentazin (perphenazine) 5 mg is used.

Cataract Nursing

Knocking the eye. The eye could be knocked by the patient himself if the sight of his other eye was poor and he was allowed to do things for himself unaided. It would be possible for the nurse to knock it in the careless turning down of the top sheet.

GENERAL NURSING CARE

Position in Bed. The patient should be on his back to prevent the pillow touching his eye. He may be lying flat or sitting up; as these patients are old it is usually more comfortable for them to be *propped up with pillows or a bed rest*. The foot of the bed can be raised on six inch bed blocks. This position makes eating easier and reduces the discomfort from flatulence.

If possible the locker and bedside table should be on the side of the unaffected eye so that any movement of the head will be towards that side.

Lifting in Bed. Although the patient is in all other respects nursed on bed rest, he is allowed to move himself if he does not do it suddenly. The usual nursing lift with the head forward would not be good for the eye. The best way is for two nurses to turn back the heavy bedclothes and then help him to sit forward, keeping his head erect. He should then support himself with his hands behind him on the bed, while the nurses rearrange the pillows; they should then help him to lift himself back. It is sudden, jerky movements which are likely to harm the eye. It will take two nurses to help him while he is in bed.

Washing. Older patients, particularly men, are not usually fond of washing, and for the first few days the less they are disturbed the better. It is therefore of importance that the patient should have had a thorough bath, including hair washing, before operation. After operation he should not be allowed to wash himself in bed; this is a difficult feat for the young with good sight and it cannot be done satisfactorily by a 'cataract' patient. There is also the slight risk of injury to the eye.

For the care of the back he should be rolled towards the side away from that of the operation.

When the patient is allowed to get out of bed washing may be done in a washing cubicle or bathroom with the patient sitting on a

Cataract Nursing

chair; it may not be quicker but the patient is much more able to help himself than when lying in bed.

Hair. The hair should be attended to when the bandage is removed for dressing the eye. If short and not easily tangled, a woman's hair may be combed after the first dressing; nothing hurts the eye so much as pulling at tangles and the nurse must use her discretion. If the hair is well plaited it may be left for three or four days, but the patient appreciates a comb put through the hair close to the head.

Shaving. Men should not be allowed to shave themselves while in hospital owing to the difficulty of doing it with poor sight and in strange surroundings. A nurse, if skilled with an electric razor, may do it for him after 48 hours.

Feeding. The patient's meals must be supervised to prevent undue movement. Surgeons vary considerably as to how long they consider it necessary for a patient to be fed. It is obviously essential if the patient has very little sight and while he is in bed; in any case a member of the staff should be at hand at meal times to give help as required. It is not easy to feed a helpless patient and especially when he is blind and also very likely to be deaf; it is wiser to allow him to have a hand on the feeder to tip it as required owing to the risk of coughing if the drink is given too fast. It is usual to allow him to hold sandwiches or cake, but not to use a spoon or fork. The imaginative nurse will add to his pleasure in the meals by remembering that he cannot see and describe the food, warning him when a mouthful is different from preceding ones and when he is approaching the end of the course.

The Diet should be light and not require much biting or chewing as movement of the jaws affects the eye: for this reason crusts, unminced meat, etc. are avoided at first.

When the patient is allowed to feed himself his tray should be carefully arranged in front of him, if possible on a bed-table. Meals in bed are not easy at any time and old people find them specially difficult.

Care at Night. Elderly patients are apt to become a little confused at night especially if they are in strange surroundings. For this reason a special nurse would be desirable for the first few nights if the patient is in a single room. It is advisable to have a shaded light over

Cataract Nursing

the bed or in the ward or room so that the nurse can notice the least restlessness.

An hypnotic drug may be necessary for the first few nights when restlessness must be avoided.

A male patient should always have a urinal within his reach.

It is sometimes advisable to tie the patient's wrists loosely with flannel bandage to the side of the bed, sufficient length being allowed for him to reach his nose on the side of the good eye. It can be explained to him that the sleeping draught may make him a little confused when he first wakes up and he may try to rub his eye before he remembers where he is.

Aperients. It does no harm to the patient to be constipated for three or four days, but if it is worrying him it may be the cause of undue restlessness. It is a good routine to give liquid paraffin or cream of magnesia as required after operation and glycerin suppositories on the third night. The aim is to avoid the straining to pass a constipated stool or, alternatively, the urgent desire following too strong an aperient. In some instances it is better to allow the use of a commode or to take the patient in a wheel chair to the lavatory, but if it is before he has been allowed to get up, the surgeon's permission must be obtained. The modern tendency is to realize the difficulty and distress of using a bedpan and the relative value of being allowed to go to the lavatory.

Smoking. This may be a problem with men. There is a real risk of fire if patients who cannot see smoke in bed; also the fumbling for matches, etc. involves a good deal of movement. If possible it should be a rule not to allow smoking until the sixth day, but if the patient is unhappy or mentally confused his pipe may be a great solace and he can be helped with the filling and lighting of it.

Getting up. After cataract operation it is ideal for a patient to be helped out of bed to sit in an arm-chair in a warm and quiet place; because hospital wards do not always provide sufficient comfortable chairs patients are sometimes reluctant to stay out of bed for most of the day. Surgeons may vary considerably as to when they judge it advisable for patients to be got up after operation and there is variation between the first and the fifth day. It should be remembered that people of over eighty often have short naps during the day

Cataract Nursing

when at home and the span of a hospital day is too long for them to keep awake. Our aim is to keep them physically and mentally active, knowing that being allowed to go to the lavatory and eating meals at a table in company of others are ways of preventing invalidism.

Visitors

One visitor who is wanted and could sit quietly by the bed, doing most of the talking and staying for about half an hour is a great pleasure to the patient. With freer visiting times it is desirable to protect patients from too many visitors in the first few days after operation.

DRESSING THE EYE AFTER OPERATION

The less disturbance to the eye the better and unless further treatment is ordered, a daily dressing is ideal. The patient will be anxious to ascertain if he can see better than before the operation. His first reaction to the regained sight depends very largely on the vision in the second eye; if that is very poor he will be rejoiced at any improvement. The immediate result of operation varies according to the spectacles previously worn. The removal of the lens has the effect of making the eye long-sighted so that a patient who was previously short-sighted will have it partly counteracted and may immediately see clearly. This effect accounts for the reports such as that a man could see to read *The Times* the first time his eye was uncovered. The immediate result also depends on factors such as slight post-operative corneal haze or soft lens matter after an extracapsular lens extraction. The patient can be reassured that he is in no way experiencing the full benefit of the operation. At this stage he may be disappointed and need encouragement. On the other hand he may feel that now all danger is over and he can relax his care, in which case the importance of the next few days must be impressed upon him.

Dressing Technique. It is usual to have individual packs of dressings.

Method. As long as the dressing is a surgically clean procedure an assistant will be required to hold the light.

The patient is prepared by removing the bandage or adhesive material and making sure that his head is fairly horizontal on the

Cataract Nursing

pillows; if it is forward it will be difficult to instil the drops and he will be more inclined to move it.

His arms should be inside the bedclothes, this will prevent him touching the sterile towel or even putting his hand to the eye. The Treatment Card should be placed where it can be seen. The strapping on the pad should be cut: if the pad is not stuck to the lids, it is better to remove it at once as a loose pad encourages a patient to put up his hand to hold it in position.

Fresh strapping should be cut and put on the side of the trolley. The assistant can make these preparations while the dresser washes her hands very thoroughly, drying them on a sterilized towel.

The dresser takes the covering towel by the under corners and arranges it by the eye covering the pillow.

The dressing packet is then opened and all the eye swabs are separated so that they may be picked up singly as required. In some hospitals, swab sticks are used so that the swab is not touched with the fingers, but it will be necessary to provide swabs also to absorb excess tears or hold lids which are slippery from ointment or Tulle Gras. The patient should be asked to keep both eyes closed until told to open them. If the pad on the eye is adherent, a swab should be taken and the tip only moistened with saline; with a pair of forceps in the other hand the pad is peeled off from above downwards, the swab steadying the lid. The pad is seldom securely stuck and a squeezing of lotion on to it results in a trickle down the cheek which invariably causes the patient to put up his hand. This pair of forceps is then discarded. At the first dressing there may be a suture holding the upper lid closed. This is inserted at operation following the paralysis of the lids by an injection into the seventh nerve. It should be cut near to the skin of the lid, the stitch drawn out and then cut near to the strapping on the cheek so that it need not be removed.

The swabbing must be done without exerting any pressure on the eye. When any discharge has been removed, it is helpful to draw down the lower lid to make sure that the eye can open and to do the same for the other eye. The patient is then asked to open both eyes; a swab held on the cheek will catch any overflow of tears that may occur when the affected eye is opened for the first time.

When the patient is used to the daylight, the assistant can be asked

Cataract Nursing

to bring the light on to the cheek first and then up to the eye, the patient having been warned.

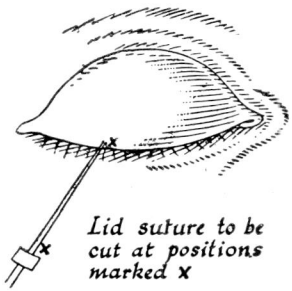

CUTTING LID SUTURE

The eye should be looked at methodically as described on page 35. The special points to notice after cataract operation are:

1. If the cornea is bright and clear.
2. If the anterior chamber has reformed.
3. If the pupil is round and central and the degree of dilatation.
4. If the section is flat and is healing without any suspicion of prolapse.

It is sometimes necessary for drops to be instilled: the eye sometimes seems a little insensitive just after operation and in this case it is easy to put in a drop. Occasionally it is hypersensitive and great care is needed to prevent the patient squeezing his eye. If a clean pad is to be applied, the patient should be asked to 'close' his eye as he will be more likely to do it gently than if told to 'shut' it. The fresh strapping should be applied with gentle pressure on the cheek and the forehead.

The second eye always requires swabbing, a point which the inexperienced nurse will forget.

Some hospitals use a Cartella shield (see page 116) strapped over the pad for added protection should the eye be touched. The disadvantage is that it requires more strapping on the face and especially with a slight growth of beard, it is not always easy to fix it securely each time the eye is inspected or dressed.

Cataract Nursing

Opportunity should be taken to attend to the patient's hair before re-applying the bandage.

When there are several eye dressings to be done consecutively it is usual to set one tray or trolley and use it for several cases. If this is done the order of the dressings must be planned so that those most recently operated upon are done first. Special care is required for an infected eye, e.g. acute conjunctivitis or dacryocystitis, and everything must be resterilized.

The following precautions must also be taken:

1. Separate dressing packs should be used for each patient.

2. If possible, containers of drops and ointment should be individual for each patient.

3. If the setting is on a tray the small receiver or paper bag for used dressings must be emptied after each dressing so that they are not carried from one patient to another.

4. The dressing round should be done quickly so that the tray does not remain in use for a long time.

Obviously the nurse must wash her hands thoroughly after each treatment.

This dressing technique differs from the usual surgical one, but the eye treatments such as drops, ointment, hot bathings, etc. are not comparable to the dressing of a surgical wound. In the hands of an intelligent and conscientious nursing staff it is a satisfactory and practical method as long as the recent operation cases and the infected eyes are dealt with on strict aseptic lines.

SUGGESTED SCHEME OF CATARACT ROUTINE FOR HOSPITAL NURSING

At the risk of repetition, a scheme of Cataract Nursing is outlined. Some recognized routine is essential in a nurse's training school. It also has a value in an eye ward in that patients will consider restrictions to be fair when they see everyone treated alike; in a men's ward this is a surprising asset in ensuring their co-operation.

When the necessity for the routine has been accepted, it must be constantly borne in mind that it is only a framework and may be varied considerably with individual patients and for different surgeons.

Cataract Nursing

Pre-operative Period.

Admitted one day before operation.

Examination of general health with special reference to chest and urine.

Thorough bath and hair wash.

Constipation may be dealt with by suppositories.

Explanation of the importance of breathing and leg exercises and of the post-operative restrictions.

Local Treatment.

Conjunctival swab taken for culture.

Antibiotic drops as ordered.

Eye lashes cut and preparation such as sac syringing and tonometry reading as ordered.

The Day of Operation.

Pre-anaesthetic treatment as ordered.

Hair arranged in two plaits.

Men shaved.

The patient's locker and bedside table moved to the side of the unaffected eye.

Observation that the culture report is satisfactory and mydriatic drops if ordered.

Dentures removed.

If the pupil is not satisfactorily dilated, the fact should be reported to the House Surgeon.

Post-operative Period.

The bed to be prepared with bedrest and at least 4 pillows.

The patient should be lifted gently from the theatre trolley. Under no circumstances must he be rolled for the removal of the trolley canvas.

It is usual for one eye only to be covered.

Instructions to the patient when he is settled in bed and is awake after the anaesthetic.

1. Not to turn on his side.
2. Not to touch his eye.
3. Not to try and reach things on his locker or table.
4. To try not to cough.

Cataract Nursing

5. To do periodic deep breathing and leg exercises.
6. To ring his bell or call for a nurse if he wants anything.

All general treatment, including speaking to him, to be done from the side of the unoperated eye if possible.

Evening Care.

Hands only to be washed.

Urinal to be given or bedpan with the help of two nurses; pillows to be made comfortable.

The light over the bed to be shaded (to be continued each night). Sedative, e.g. Soneryl.

First Day.

Morning wash, hands and around mouth only; back powdered with the patient lifted and not rolled.

Mouth rinsed carefully.

Patient made comfortable and bed straightened by two nurses.

Eye dressed by the surgeon or sister (many surgeons like it left until the second day).

Helped to sit out of bed in a chair for a short time.

Evening wash, hands and face, back with spirit and powder.

Second Day Onwards.

Gradual mobilization, aiming at full activity by the fifth day.

Men may be shaved with an electric razor if the condition of the eye is satisfactory.

Mild aperient if necessary.

The time at which the patient is discharged from the ward will vary considerably according to the condition of the eye, home conditions and the practice of the individual surgeon.

Advice to the patient on discharge.

To be careful not to knock or damage the eye.

Activities such as strenuous housework or gardening should not be undertaken. Not to be out of doors in a cold wind. It is inadvisable to wash the hair for a week or two.

To report to the doctor if the eye becomes painful or inflamed.

COMPLICATIONS
Local Complications

It is essential for a nurse to be alert to the complications which

Cataract Nursing

could occur. With continual stress on early mobilization after operation, and with a dilution of trained nurses working in the wards, it is particularly important that complications are recognized as early as possible.

Post-operative Iritis. The symptoms and signs are, pain 'round the eye', photophobia, a red eye, a small pupil and muddy iris.

The condition is more common in diabetics and may be very resistant to treatment which consists of mydriatics, local cortisone, heat and dark glasses. Analgesic drugs will usually be necessary.

Hyphaema. This is the condition of blood between the cornea and the iris. When it occurs the anterior chamber is full of blood and a little may trickle down the cheek, but after some hours it sinks to the bottom and is then described according to the level, e.g. total, a third full, a crescent. The haemorrhage is not always sufficient to fill the anterior chamber.

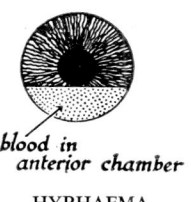

HYPHAEMA

Hyphaema is due to bleeding from the iris or the edges of the incision and may be spontaneous or the result of a knock. It is usually accompanied by some pain and the patient will notice that he cannot see through it. It may re-absorb in a day or two or may remain for some time; in the latter case, there is some risk of secondary glaucoma or of some staining of the cornea. The treatment is rest, to prevent further haemorrhage; heat may be ordered and can conveniently be applied with an electric warmer; the movement involved in hot bathing would not be balanced by the value of the heat.

Pain may be acute and should be relieved by codeine or other drugs.

Diabetic patients are very much more liable to hyphaema.

Prolapsed Iris. The iris prolapses through the incision and appears as a black bead. The pupil is drawn up towards it.

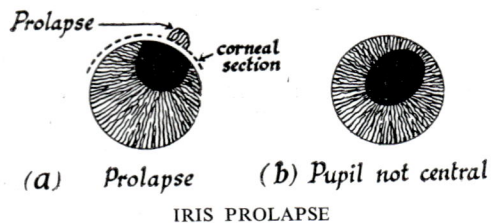

(a) Prolapse   *(b)* Pupil not central

IRIS PROLAPSE

The shape of the pupil should be carefully noted daily and slight alteration should arouse anxiety.

The prolapse may be present at the first dressing with no obvious symptoms: the surgeon sometimes has difficulty in replacing the iris at the end of the operation and when it occurs in these cases it could not have been prevented by nursing care.

The iris can prolapse at any time during the first week, but it is more common in the first few days and may follow squeezing of the eye or a slight knock or violent coughing or vomiting. There is usually sharp pain at the time of the accident.

Treatment consists of further operation, Replacement or Abscission of Iris Prolapse. It should not affect the eye as far as the sight is concerned, but there is often some post-operative iritis.

Septic Infection. This is fortunately rare, but it may occur in patients with low resistance to infection, as the very old or where there is intercurrent disease. Early signs are, a yellowish appearance of the incision, hazy cornea, a red eye and chemosis.

Chemotherapy has considerably improved the prognosis.

General Complications

Retention of Urine. This is a common complication in men and is usually due to an enlarged prostate gland. If the patient has been given a urinal to use in bed before operation it will be a useful indication if he has difficulty and allows the fact to be reported to the surgeon beforehand. If retention occurs in the first few days afterwards, the surgeon will usually give permission for him to be helped to stand out of bed as the alternative to catheterization which involves the greater disturbance. It is important to deal with the matter before the bladder becomes overdistended.

Cataract Nursing

Chest Complications. These include bronchitis, pleurisy, hypostatic pneumonia and pulmonary emboli. There is much less risk of them when the surgeon allows patients to be got out of bed soon after operation. Should the patient have to be kept at rest for a longer time it is important to teach him deep breathing exercises, if possible with the supervision of a physiotherapist.

Femoral thrombosis. The risk of thrombosis is reduced by leg exercises and by getting out of bed and walking. The early signs are tenderness of the calf and slight pyrexia.

Post-operative Mental Confusion or Mania. It is not uncommon for these patients to become slightly confused at night, but fortunately mania is rare. The danger to the eye is from the restlessness, but a surprising number survive with useful vision; in fact, it makes the inexperienced nurse question the necessity for the usual care. The condition should be reported in the slightest form, such as unusual volubility or a searching for things in the bed. The surgeon will usually allow the patient to sit in an arm-chair with altogether as little restriction as possible. The patient is often sent home a few days after operation.

The violent cases must be treated as they would if arising at any other time and they also may recover with a useful eye.

A ward sister's round can usefully include the following observations of each patient: has the temperature been above normal? is urine passed easily? has he any cough? has he any discomfort in his legs? The patient's visitors can often provide useful information when commenting that his conversation or behaviour is odd or that he is extremely anxious about his bowels. When patients were kept in bed in a ward a nurse found it easier to observe stools or urine output or how food was taken, but now we have more of a problem and must maintain vigilance in the changed circumstances.

AFTER CATARACT

This is the condition which occurs when opacity of the remaining lens capsule interferes with clear vision, and it is often the case after removal of lens by the extra-capsular operation. The small operation of *Capsulotomy*, the tearing of a central hole in the capsule,

Cataract Nursing

is done with a discission needle and is commonly termed 'Needling'. This is usually performed a few weeks after the first operation when the eye is quiet.

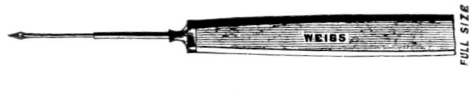

BOWMAN'S NEEDLE

Capsulotomy is an intra-ocular operation, but the incision is only the width of the blade of the needle.

Possible complications are iritis and rise of intra-ocular tension due to the disturbance of residual soft lens matter.

Cataract Spectacles. The prescribing of spectacles is usually delayed until the eye has become completely quiet so that further change will not be necessary. When the sight of the other eye is poor, temporary glasses are sometimes given at once. Because of their thickness, cataract glasses are correspondingly heavy and patients sometimes ask for plastic lenses to reduce the weight. Plastic lenses are more expensive and scratch very easily. All glasses should be put down so that the centre of the lens is not touching the table and this is especially necessary with plastic cataract glasses.

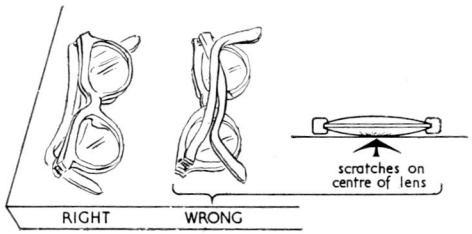

THE RIGHT AND WRONG WAY TO PUT GLASSES DOWN ON A TABLE

The glasses are difficult to use at first owing to the strength of the convex lenses and the patient is frequently disappointed when he wears them and is unable to see as well as when he was tested. He should return to the optician to make certain that the frames are

Cataract Nursing

correctly adjusted and then be advised to persevere for a week or two. If they continue to be uncomfortable he should see the surgeon.

The following two pamphlets have been written for distribution to patients following a doctor's explanation to them.

The first pamphlet aims at explaining to patients who are about to have a cataract operation that their new glasses may take a little while, and some perseverance, before they can see well again. It is a fact that a patient who has very poor vision before the operation can usually get accustomed to the new glasses more quickly than one who sees fairly well with his better eye, and this is one reason for surgeons deciding not to operate too early.

'EYESIGHT AND SPECTACLES AFTER CATARACT OPERATION

Sometime in the near future you will have a cataract removed from one eye. Once that is done you have an excellent chance of obtaining better vision in that eye. However, since being forewarned is forearmed it will help you to know the following:

1. The cataract is really the lens of your eye which has become cloudy and just as a camera needs a lens so does your eye. Having removed the cataract, i.e. the lens, a substitute lens is placed in a spectacle frame in front of your eye. *Thus you will only obtain clear vision when wearing your spectacles.*

2. Because the eye takes a few weeks to settle down following the operation, spectacles will not be prescribed immediately. Don't be depressed if you don't see clearly immediately following the operation. Clear vision will only come when you have your spectacles. These are normally prescribed three to six weeks after the operation.

3. The spectacles are usually heavier than those to which you are accustomed. You will soon get used to this.

4. Unlike a camera the eye uses the lens in order to focus. When the lens is removed from your eye this ability to focus is lost. Thus you will require two pairs of spectacles—one for close work and one for distance.

5. Because the glass in the spectacles needs to be thick you only

Cataract Nursing

see clearly through the centre of it. This results in some loss of side vision or what we call field of vision. Initially you may find this troublesome when going downstairs or when stepping off the kerb. You must learn to turn and bend your head where previously you turned your eyes. Turning your eyes only will result in distortion because you will be looking through the edge of the glass—*so learn to turn your head and look straight through your glasses.*

6. Until you adapt to your new glasses you will experience difficulty in estimating the relative position of objects and you will experience some distortion as you move towards a large object such as a door. If you persevere you will soon overcome these difficulties.

7. If the cataract is removed from only one eye you can no longer use both eyes together (just as you would not expect to obtain the same picture with two cameras—one with a lens and one without) because you will not get the same sized picture in each eye. It may be necessary to cloud the spectacle glass in front of one eye to prevent you seeing double.

Finally, remember that many hundreds of patients have this operation each year, and that all soon adapt themselves.'

The second pamphlet deals with the uncommon problem of cataract in one eye only; this may occur after an accident which results in a traumatic cataract. It is usual for cataract to develop gradually in both eyes, but one advances more quickly than the other and the surgeon delays the decision to operate until sight is insufficient for what the patient wants to do. For example, a patient might see to get about quite well but long to be able to read again, and it would be very helpful to him to have his worse eye operated on and use reading glasses for that eye but continue to use his other eye for all other purposes.

'CATARACT IN ONE EYE

You have a cataract in one of your eyes, and these notes have been written to enable you to understand the implications of this.

A cataract is not a skin on the eye to be peeled off at operation but rather the normal lens of the eye has become clouded and sometimes completely opaque so that you cannot see out into the world properly

Cataract Nursing

with that eye, nor can the examining oculist see in. Your other eye is normal, and it is on this account that a problem arises as to the best line of treatment.

The only way in which it is possible to make you see better with your bad eye is by removing the lens of the eye entirely. This is done at operation and leaves the eye rather like a camera without part of its lens system, so that the vision afterwards is very blurred (rather like looking at things under water).

Now in order to make the eye see again clearly we can give a strong lens in the glasses, but this lens must necessarily be worn in front of the eye whereas the natural lens was inside the eye, and the result of this is that the eye sees things much larger than before (about 20 per cent magnification).

It will therefore be seen that it is not possible to use this eye with the normal eye on the other side, otherwise a very severe form of double vision is produced; therefore, in your case the possible alternatives are as follows:

(a) To take no action at all.

(b) To remove the lens of the eye at operation, but not to give the necessary glasses to make you see clearly with that eye. The advantage of this is twofold. First, that you would be much more aware of people standing on the same side as your bad eye, and secondly, you would have the eye in reserve in case of an accident to or cataract developing in the other eye.

(c) To fit a contact lens on the eye we have operated on. This lens is worn under the eyelids and on the front of the eyeball, and because it is so close to the eye this eye sees things much more normally, and the two eyes can be used together. As you can imagine, contact lenses have to be most carefully made and take a lot of getting used to, but this is not insuperable. Many people in their seventies have been fitted successfully with contact lenses.

It is these three possibilities which form the basis of any discussion we may have as to the future of your eyes.'

ARTIFICIAL INTRA-OCULAR LENSES

In cataract operations there has been an attempt to replace the lens removed at operation by insertion into the eye of a lens made of

Cataract Nursing

an inert plastic material similar to Perspex. This lens has the refractive power of the human lens but obviously it cannot accommodate to focus near objects and reading glasses will be necessary. The great advantage is that the heavy convex spectacle lens will not be necessary; these glasses magnify the image unnaturally and only give clear sight through the centre of the lens. For these reasons the patient gets distorted vision if one eye has been operated on and the second has not; with an intra-ocular lens both eyes can be used together to give normal binocular vision.

There are different types of intra-ocular implants; one type is similar in shape to the human lens and is inserted behind the pupil in the position where it would normally lie. Another type is placed in the anterior chamber so that it is between the cornea and the iris. These lenses are ordered for each patient to his individual requirements and are usually inserted at a subsequent operation when the eye has settled down after the lens extraction; the eye often reacts with some degree of post-operative iritis which should clear up in a week or two. If the eye does not tolerate the lens, it is possible to remove it. An anterior chamber implant has been used for the correction of high myopia and for this purpose it would be inserted into the eye with the normal lens in position. The advance in contact lens techniques has partly replaced the need for intra-ocular lenses in cases of monocular aphakia and high myopia.

The post-operative nursing care is similar to that already described. Corneoscleral sutures may be inserted and these will be removed by the surgeon usually about a week after operation.

Recent experience is showing that the intra-ocular lenses are not well tolerated in all eyes and their value is not as great as was hoped.

9

SURGICAL NURSING (continued)

CORNEAL GRAFTING

Corneal grafting (Keratoplasty) is the operation in which a portion of opaque cornea is replaced by a graft from a healthy eye. The graft can be of the full thickness of the cornea, a *'penetrating'* graft or it can be of the superficial layers when it is called a *'partial thickness'* or *'lamellar'* graft; the lamellar graft is used where the opacity is only in the surface of the cornea or when it is considered advisable to do a larger preliminary lamellar graft to be followed later on by a small penetrating one. The graft is usually circular in shape, from four to ten millimetres in diameter, five or six millimetres being an average size for a full thickness one.

The aim of corneal grafting is usually to improve the sight of an eye in which central corneal scars prevent the rays of light entering the pupil; the scarring may be due to a variety of causes, e.g. corneal ulcers, keratitis associated with tuberculosis or acne rosacea, corneal dystrophy, etc. and the prognosis of the operation depends in some degree on the original cause. In a large number of cases the graft remains transparent and perfect sight is restored. The lamellar graft may be used therapeutically for an ulcer which fails to respond to other treatment or for a severe corneal burn.

The graft may be taken from an eye in which the cornea is healthy but the eye was excised for other reasons, for example, because it was blind and painful; the eye would be used within an hour of removal and is usually thought to be the best material. The more usual source is the eye which has been removed as soon as possible after a patient has died; it is then stored in a refrigerator and used within the next

Surgical Nursing

few days. Research is being carried out to determine whether there are any factors, similar to blood groups, which control the suitability of grafting material and to ascertain the best conditions for storage of the donor eyes. The legal position regarding the taking of these eyes varies in different countries but, in Britain, The Corneal Grafting Act, 1952, allows the eyes of a deceased person to be used for therapeutic purposes unless he or his surviving relatives have objected to it. The practice is increasing whereby a person bequeaths his eyes for corneal grafting purposes after his death. The Royal National Institute for the Blind have specially prepared forms for the purpose and are very grateful to prospective donors who should be sure that their nearest relative knows of their intention so that the appropriate steps may be taken as soon as possible after death.

The nursing care follows the principles of that for any intra-ocular operation. The preparation is as for cataract operation except that the pupil will not require dilatation. The operation may be done under local anaesthesia but a general anaesthetic is advisable for a very nervous patient or in case of nystagmus where the eye cannot be kept still: a few patients react to a bright light with reflex sneezing and this would make operation under local anaesthetic impossible; a nurse's observation on such a point can be of much value to the surgeon.

The post-operative care should be explained to the patient. Much that is written in the popular press leads patients to expect that their sight will be perfect as soon as the eye is uncovered; this is misleading as the sutures or corneal covering will certainly obscure the

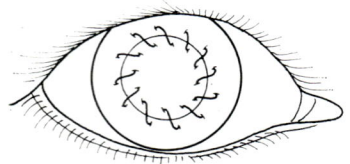
CONTINUOUS SUTURE

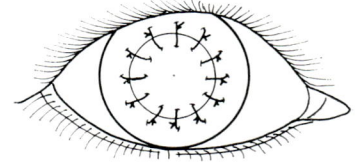
INTERRUPTED SUTURES

CORNEAL GRAFT SUTURES
N.B. In the drawing, the sutures have been enlarged for clarity

Surgical Nursing

vision in most cases and the full degree of improvement is not attained until the eye has completely recovered from the operation. *The chief complication* to be guarded against is displacement of the graft. At operation the graft is held in place with sutures or with one of various types of corneal cap; whatever method is used the aim is to allow the graft to heal with its edges exactly flush with the surrounding cornea. If the graft tilts, aqueous may leak out and the iris can become adherent between the edge of the graft and its bed; this anterior synechia is a predisposing cause of opacity of the graft. The later complication is a gradually increasing opacity and vascularity of the graft: treatment with local steroid drugs will help to prevent vascularization occurring, and recent advances in tissue typing ensure that less grafts, which have apparently taken well, become opaque at a later date.

Nursing care is aimed at keeping the eye still so that healing takes place with the graft in perfect position. Either one or both eyes may be bandaged for several days. The nursing routine can be as that for cataract operation (see page 139) with the following differences. After cataract operation it is essential to look at the eye to make sure that the section is healing with the iris in place; after corneal graft it is important to note whether the graft is clear and its surface flush with the surrounding cornea, also the depth of the anterior chamber and pupil size should be noted. Many of these patients have had prolonged corneal disease and are specially liable to sensitivity to drugs such as atropine or to Vaseline gauze or even to cotton wool. Any sign of such irritation should be reported immediately so that appropriate treatment can be given. Atropine is an important part of the treatment as it is prophylactic against iritis and also ensures that the pupil is larger than the size of the graft thus preventing anterior synechiae. A local antibiotic such as penicillin and local steroids such as Betnesol are usually ordered. The corneal sutures may be left in for several weeks and will then be removed by the surgeon.

The surface of the graft remains insensitive for several weeks and while this is the case the eye must be kept covered when out of doors in rough weather.

If the graft is not quite flat, a firm pad and bandage will be ordered

Surgical Nursing

and if the condition does not improve a tarsorrhaphy may be done; this is a minor operation in which the edges of the lids are sewn together to protect the cornea. The tarsorrhaphy may be left for several months and when opened there will be no deformity or scarring of the lids.

GLAUCOMA

Glaucoma is a condition of increased tension in the eyeball. It can be due to various causes; the rigid sclera and cornea will not stretch and therefore any increase in the contents of the eyeball, such as a rapidly growing tumour or a haemorrhage inside the eye, would cause a rise of tension. In these cases the condition would be of secondary glaucoma, but the most common problem is that of glaucoma which arises without obvious reason. This primary glaucoma is an eye condition the cause of which is still not fully understood and much research in connection with it is being done at the present time; it is associated with a defective drainage of aqueous fluid. The aqueous is a body fluid similar to lymph and it is continually secreted by the ciliary body and circulates in the part of the eye which is between the lens and the cornea and it drains away into tiny canals which join the venous capillaries. The position of the drainage canals is between the outer edge of the iris and the junction of the cornea and sclera, and this area is known as the drainage angle of the anterior chamber.

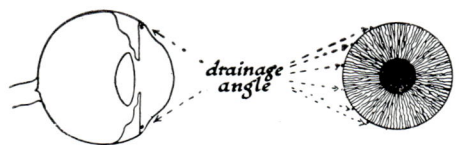

DRAINAGE ANGLE

As the eyeball cannot swell to accommodate any increase in its contents the tension rises and the weakest part gives way; this is the optic disc at the back of the eye where the nerve fibres from the retina leave the eye to form the optic nerve. As the optic disc becomes pressed backwards it deepens and the nerve fibres are subjected to pressure as they pass over the edge of the 'cupped' disc. Prolonged

Surgical Nursing

pressure will cause atrophy of these nerves from the retina with resulting blindness. The particular form of blindness which it causes is loss of visual field. While the central vision, as tested on a test type of letters (see p. 22) may be good, there is progressive contraction of the field of vision and enlargement of the normal blind spot. These changes may pass unnoticed by the patient, especially if only one eye is affected, but the very serious fact is that the field losses are irreversible and they may gradually encroach on the central vision so that one eye may be virtually blind before specialist advice is sought. One reason why glaucoma may not be recognized is that there is often no pain in the eye, and it is a disease that is frequently found by a doctor, or an optician during a routine eye test for glasses; an optician is not qualified to diagnose or treat eye disease but he is trained to recognize a departure from the normal and he plays a valuable part in our health service by referring patients to their own doctors for expert investigation of suspicious conditions.

Glaucoma is fortunately a disease of middle and old age but as the expected span of life gets longer so a condition which causes blindness becomes an increasing problem. As research results in further understanding of the pathology and causes of glaucoma so the treatment can be expected to change, but at present much stress is laid on early diagnosis and on continuous supervision so that deterioration can be checked as soon as possible. There is a commendable trend in medical care to explain the situation to a patient and advise him to ask for a further appointment if he thinks it necessary, but glaucoma is an exception and it is most desirable to repeat the relevant tests at regular intervals even if no symptoms are present.

Glaucoma Tests

The tests most usually done are those for measuring the intraocular tension (see p. 96), and those for recording fields of vision (see p. 26). Other tests are variations of these and certain measures which are sometimes taken to provoke a rise of tension to confirm the diagnosis in borderline cases. In an ophthalmic hospital it is usual to have special glaucoma clinics when the appointments are spaced to allow longer periods for the tests. In addition to tonometry

Surgical Nursing

with a Schiötz tonometer (see p. 96) there are other instruments for recording intra-ocular tension which are used by the doctor. An applanation tonometer is used in conjunction with a slit-lamp and an electronic instrument is also used.

Repeated tonometry or phasing

The normal intra-ocular tension shows a diurnal variation with a maximum in the early morning, and in certain types of glaucoma the tension may be raised for periods during the day. For this reason it is sometimes valuable to admit a patient for tonometry readings at frequent intervals, for example three-hourly, throughout the day and night. The readings are recorded as a graph and may be repeated on different treatments until satisfactory control is maintained, or it is considered advisable to operate as the only means of controlling the glaucoma. Because of the frequency of the tests the corneal surface should be lubricated after each tonometry reading and it is usual to use guttae Paroleine.

Tonography

Another variation of tonometry tests is tonography which is done to ascertain the rate of outflow of aqueous fluid. In a normal eye the pressure of a tonometer resting on the eye for four minutes will increase the drainage of aqueous and the tension falls steadily. In open-angle glaucoma the tension does not fall. To carry out the test the patient must be lying comfortably on a couch with his eye thoroughly anaesthetized with drops such as Decicain. The doctor sits at the head of the couch and uses a tonometer with various weights because the standard outflow charts show graphs for use with particular weights. A stop-watch is used to check the time and the doctor holds the tonometer on the eye for four minutes, watching the scale for the expected fall in pressure.

Gonioscopy

This is a method of examining the angle of the anterior chamber with a gonioscope.

This instrument is used in conjunction with a slit-lamp; it is a type of contact lens which contains a mirror that deflects the light into

Surgical Nursing

the opposite angle and allows this illuminated angle to be seen with the magnification provided by the slit-lamp. To use a simile, it is as though one could see under the rim of a watch case which covers the outer edge of the watch glass and hides the 'angle' of the space in which the hands move round.

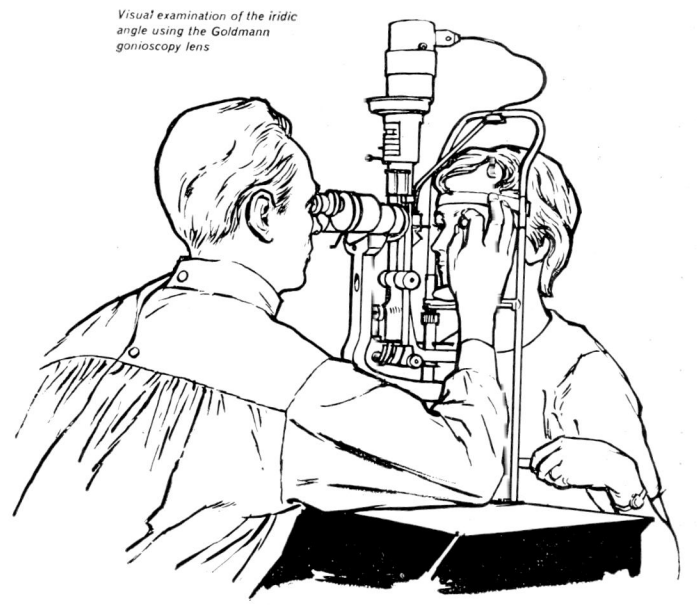

Visual examination of the iridic angle using the Goldmann gonioscopy lens

In preparation for gonioscopy local anaesthetic drops are instilled and a fluid will be required to fill the lens; this fluid can be normal saline or Methocel and should be in a drop bottle. After use the gonioscope should be rinsed under cold water and dried with a soft tissue; the plastic material of which it is made can be damaged by disinfectants or heat or by scratching the surface if dried on a cloth. A box lined with sponge rubber is provided for its safe keeping when not in use.

PROVOCATIVE TESTS

These are various tests which may be done to provoke a rise in

Surgical Nursing

tension when the diagnosis is doubtful. These tests will be negative in normal eyes but a positive result may be of much value where the result of other investigations is inconclusive.

Dark Room Test

The basis of this test is that the pupil will dilate in the dark so that the periphery of the iris takes up more space and tends to block the drainage angle, causing a rise in tension. The test is of value in closed angle glaucoma. The patient is put into a dark room for one hour and a comparison is made of the tension reading before and afterwards; the patient should not go to sleep as there is a relaxation factor associated with sleep which would confuse the result of the test. A rise of tension of 5 mm. Hg. or more is significant.

Nursing points for the carrying out of the test are:

1. Explanation to the patient of how long the test will take and suggestion that he goes to the toilet so that he will not be uncomfortable during the hour.

2. The room must be completely blacked out and there should be an 'Engaged' sign for the door so that other staff do not go in and out.

3. The patient should sit in a comfortable chair but not lie on a couch or bed when he might not be able to keep awake.

4. A few people are truly claustrophobic and this test might cause distress; if this is the case the doctor should be consulted and if it is very desirable to carry out the test someone might sit with the patient or a transistor radio might help. In any case the patient should be assured that staff will be at hand and someone will make sure that he is all right about half-time.

5. A cup of tea should not be offered during the hour as the fluid intake could affect the test.

6. The same tonometer must be used for both readings and they should be done by the same nurse.

It has been remarked in jest that conditions in a cinema in congenial company would be ideal for a dark-room test.

Water Drinking Test

In this test the variation in tension is recorded when a patient who had had no fluid for some hours then drinks a large quantity in a short time. In normal eyes there is an increase in tension of a few millimetres within half an hour and then a return to the previous reading within an hour. An increase of more than 5 mm would be suspicious, especially if it was associated with a slow return to the previous level.

Method. The test is usually carried out in the early morning. The patient must not have anything to drink from before midnight. The tension is recorded and the patient must then drink one litre of water within five minutes. The tension is recorded at quarter-hourly intervals for one hour, and if by then it has not returned to the previous level the readings should be continued.

Nursing points. If the patient is an out-patient it can be discussed with him how early he would like to attend so that he is not without fluid for too long. He should be told how long the test will take. If he is using miotic drops he should put them in as usual that morning. On arrival he should be asked if he has had a cup of tea or anything to drink, because it would be a waste of time if he had misunderstood or forgotten the instructions. After taking the first tonometry reading he should be sat down with the water in a jug and a clock in view so that he knows how much time there is to complete the drinking. He may need encouragement as it is a large quantity for someone not used to drinking water. If he is very old or of very small stature it may be wise to reduce the quantity a little as long as the exact volume is recorded. Further readings at quarter-hourly intervals must be taken by the same nurse. Because there must be a couch free and the nurse available at the exact times it is often not convenient to arrange for this test while a busy clinic is being held, and equally it may not be possible for a ward patient if there is only one nurse on duty and all the patients are just waking up and requiring attention.

Mydriatic test

This test compares the tension of an eye with a normal pupil with the same eye after the pupil has been dilated with mydriatic drops. In a normal eye there is little variation, but in an eye predisposed to glaucoma the tension may increase to above normal limits and then fail to respond to miotic drops which normally counteract the mydriatic ones. The test is of value in closed angle glaucoma.

Nursing points. This test is often carried out without being specifically mentioned, because a tension reading is frequently required both before and after mydriatic drops. If glaucoma is suspected a very mild mydriatic is used, for example, cocaine drops, with the idea that it will be easier to counteract them if the tension rises. One drop only should be instilled and should not be repeated if the pupil fails to dilate. If a mydriatic test has been done it is usual for the nurse to be asked to keep the patient under observation until the pupils are fully contracted.

Acute Glaucoma

A patient suffering from narrow angle glaucoma may have an attack of acute glaucoma and also the acute phase occurs secondarily to other eye conditions such as acute iridocyclitis or as a postoperative complication, or following certain eye injuries. The acute attack of raised tension is one of the most painful eye conditions and is associated with nausea and vomiting and extreme misery. The pain is in the eye, but also in the surrounding area and it is typical to see such a patient sitting with a handkerchief over his eye and his head supported by his hand. During the examination of the eye typical features will be the sudden reduction in vision and a very red eye which is tender to touch. The loss of sight is mainly due to oedema of the cornea, and as an aid to diagnosis this oedema can be temporarily cleared by eye drops of glycerin, either pure or 50 per cent. The clearing will allow examination with a slit lamp and an ophthalmoscope. Glycerin drops are painful and should be preceded by local anaesthetic ones, such as Decicain. A patient with acute glaucoma will usually require admission with a view to further investigations, treatment, and possibly operation. The immediate treatment aims at reducing the very high tension by miotic drops given very frequently and by Diamox given intramuscularly or intravenously. Fentazin is sometimes given to control the nausea which may be aggravated by eserine drops. Glycerol may be given by mouth for its dehydrating action. At one time aperients such as calomel followed by salts, and retention enemas of magnesium sul-

Surgical Nursing

phate were given with the intention of dehydrating the body. Ocular congestion was treated by local heat and the application of leeches over the outer orbital ridge. Once the cause of the acute attack has been established the treatment will be of the underlying primary glaucoma or of the secondary cause. If the tension cannot be controlled by treatment, the operation of iridectomy is performed.

Treatment of Primary Glaucoma

Primary glaucoma is now divided into two categories depending on whether the drainage angle is narrow or closed or whether it is open, but the treatment in both kinds aims at preventing loss of field of vision by controlling the tension. The toleration of eyes to rise in tension varies considerably and it is found that some patients with a tension of below 25 mm Hg will progressively lose visual field, while others with a regular tension of over 30 mm Hg retain their fields. This is stressed because nurses may feel that there should be a definite level above which patients must not be allowed to remain, but the recent tendency is to watch the central fields very carefully if the tension is high, but not to operate unless the field is being lost.

Medical means of reducing intra-ocular tension are by drops which keep the pupil small and by drugs which reduce the secretion of aqueous fluid. The commonly used miotic drops are eserine and pilocarpine. It can be appreciated that the smaller the pupil the thinner the iris will be and it, therefore, gives more space for drainage of aqueous at the angle of the anterior chamber.

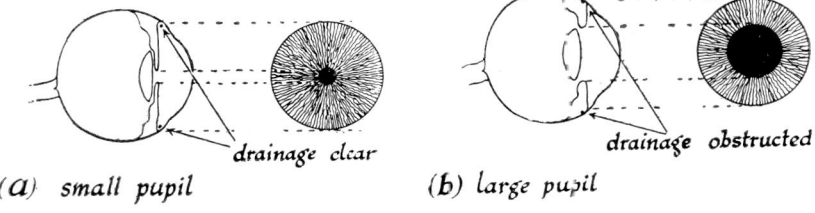

(a) small pupil — drainage clear
(b) large pupil — drainage obstructed

The miotic drops have other beneficial effects in addition to assisting drainage by a small pupil. Other drugs are also used in the form of drops for glaucoma, for example, an epinephrine solution which is thought to decrease the rate of aqueous production: it is of particular value if the patient has some cataract because it does not contract the pupil. Whatever treatment is given, regular examinations are essential to ensure that the glaucoma continues to be controlled. If medical treatment is inadequate surgery is considered. The age of the patient is an important consideration because the surgeon has to aim at preserving useful sight for as long as it will be required, and if one eye is well controlled in a patient of over 85 years there would not be serious anxiety about a deterioration in the other eye. Unfortunately, the man or woman of under 50 years is often much more difficult to treat, and if there is a strong family history of glaucoma which resulted in blindness the surgeon is very hesitant to operate. If surgery has been decided on, the surgeon explains very carefully to the patient that the operation cannot improve his sight, but is aimed at preventing it becoming worse.

The operations are undertaken to secure artificial drainage of aqueous, they include *trephining*, *sclerotomy* and *iridencleisis*. Trephining is fairly usual and the nursing care is similar in each case.

TREPHINING OPERATION (for Chronic or Subacute Glaucoma)

In this operation a disc, 1·5 mm or 2 mm in diameter, is removed from the corneoscleral margin; this hole communicates with the outer edge of the anterior chamber and because its surface is covered by conjunctiva, the aqueous drains through the hole and is absorbed by the conjunctival blood-vessels. The flap of conjunctiva is sutured with two or three silk stitches.

Nursing. This is as for an intra-ocular operation; the routine is a little less rigid than for a cataract as the incision of the eyeball is smaller and therefore there is less risk of complications. On the other hand, the fact that the eye was subjected to increased tension may make the surgeon's work more difficult.

Special nursing points

1. These patients are often reluctant to have an operation, being frightened that they may lose the little sight they have: if the surgeon has advised operation he will be keen to do it, and the line of argument must be that this holds out the best hope of retaining the present

Surgical Nursing

amount of vision, which would otherwise deteriorate irrevocably. In fact, the prognosis must be guarded, as in the most skilful hands operations are not always permanently successful.

2. The pupil should not be dilated before operation.

3. One eye only will be covered after operation.

4. The position in bed should be lying on the back with as many pillows as desired.

5. During the dressing of the eye it is important to note the depth of the anterior chamber which may remain very shallow for some days.

6. It is usual for atropine drops to be ordered to the operated eye; there is no risk of increased tension for some days and the mydriatic is prophylactic against post-operative iritis. Eserine or pilocarpine may be ordered to the other eye and this is the occasion when a mistake would be very serious if atropine was put into the wrong eye. Therefore a witness for the drops is strongly advisable for staff who are in training.

7. Some surgeons order gentle *massage* to the eyeball during the post-operative period. This is to encourage drainage through the trephine hole and is carried out by palpation on the sclera above the hole; it is done through the upper lid. The patient is asked to look down, and the tips of the two first fingers are placed on the lid so that the eyeball may be gently pressed with each alternately. The technique is similar to feeling the tension of the eye, but in this case the dimpling is repeated about a dozen times. The massage may be done two or three times a day and the surgeon may want the patient taught to do it for himself.

8. The conjunctival stitches are usually removed about the fifth day; they are high under the upper lid and can be difficult to pick up

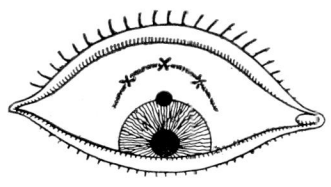

CONJUNCTIVAL FLAP

Surgical Nursing

unless the patient looks well down; it is easier to have an assistant to hold the lid rather than to insert a speculum.

Complications. (These are seldom serious.)

1. Aqueous may leak from the wound resulting in a persistently shallow anterior chamber.

2. Choroidal detachment; this usually becomes re-attached in a comparatively short time and need not give rise to anxiety.

Perforating Wound of Eye

The nursing will obviously depend on the extent of the injury. An eye which is suspected of having sustained serious damage should be very gently opened as pressure on the eye might increase an iris prolapse or vitreous loss. There is often comparatively little pain but the patient is usually frightened and shocked. He should be resting on a comfortable chair or couch until he has been examined by the doctor. Admission to hospital is always necessary and immediate operation will be performed. If it is a child the parents often ask 'He has not lost his sight, has he?' If the doctor is not available to speak to them the nurse can explain that it is not possible to know the effect of the accident at once and she can usually reassure them that his other eye is unharmed. A boy will often shield his friend who threw the dart or shot the gun, and the history given of falling and knocking his eye can be very misleading. An X-ray will usually be taken to exclude an intra-ocular foreign body. A perforating wound very often injures the lens of the eye causing a traumatic cataract so that the vision is often much reduced. Very many of these injuries are the subject of legal action and the casualty notes of the history of the accident and condition on admission are very important, as the doctor who first saw the patient is likely to have left the hospital by the date of a court case.

Pre-operative Care

Any cleansing of the eyelids and surrounding area should be done particularly gently, and in the case of a small child it might be better to leave it until he has been anaesthetized. The eye-lashes will be cut in the theatre with care that no loose lashes fall into the wound.

The operation may include excision of some prolapsed tissue followed by suture of the corneal or scleral wound and of the conjunc-

Surgical Nursing

tiva. If an intra-ocular foreign body was seen on X-ray it would be removed by an electro-magnet (see p. 196) if it was of magnetic material. Pieces of glass or plastic do not show on X-ray and are very difficult to find and remove from inside an eye. Unless the eye is very badly contused most surgeons try to repair the perforating wound with the intention of watching the eye carefully for the next days and weeks, hoping that a little useful sight can be saved even in the worst injuries. There is a danger of a sympathetic iritis occurring in the second eye and the risk of it makes a surgeon hesitate to continue treatment of an injured eye which has barely perception of light in it and little hope of improvement. If the injured eye settles down with no serious inflammation it will still be examined frequently and then at weekly intervals for a month or two after the patient has been sent home, to ensure that sympathetic iritis does not develop.

The post-operative nursing is similar to that for cataract operations. The local complications to be observant for are iritis, hyphaema, secondary glaucoma, and intra-ocular infection. Any discomfort, sensitivity to light or slight inflammation of the second eye should be reported to the doctor immediately as they might be symptoms of sympathetic iritis and it would be more likely if the onset were ten days or more after the accident. Any sutures would be removed by the doctor or on his instructions; for a small child an anaesthetic might be given to remove them and examine both eyes thoroughly.

If the injured eye settles down and heals well there may still be a traumatic cataract which might be removed at a later date.

RETINAL DETACHMENT OR SEPARATION

If the retina becomes detached from the choroid, fluid collects between them and the detachment increases in extent. Its result is loss of vision in the eye. The condition is more common in myopic eyes when it is often spontaneous, but may follow a blow on the eye; unfortunately it is sometimes bilateral. Detachment may be caused by a tumour of the choroid which strips off the retina.

The condition seldom rights itself; the older treatment was rest in bed, but now it is recognized that operation provides the best hope of a cure.

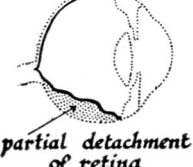
partial detachment of retina

RETINAL DETACHMENT

Cryo therapy is used where there is a hole in the retina, but little or no subretinal fluid. The frozen tip of the cryo probe is applied to the sclera over the site of the hole, causing adhesion of the tissues of the wall of the eye.

Photo coagulation is a method of aiming to seal off the retinal hole by 'light' burns; in this operation the light rays are directed through the pupil on to the affected area of the retina.

Scleral resection may be performed when the retinal detachment is associated with high myopia or aphakia. In this operation the aim is to shorten the eyeball thereby relaxing the tension on the retina; a narrow band of sclera is resected for half the circumference of the eye, the other half being done at a later date if necessary.

Encircling Band Operation. This is performed when there are several weak areas in the retina and aims at constricting the eyeball by putting a band of silicone around the circumference at the equator and pulling it slightly tight so that the eye is altered from a spherical to a slightly hour-glass shape. Because a sphere has the largest volume for its surface area, this procedure will reduce the volume of the eye thus facilitating the replacement of the retina. The foreign body effect produced on the choroid by the tightened string will irritate the choroid in the region of the band causing a little choroidal reaction which encourages the retina to adhere to it in the same way as would follow the application of diathermy or cautery. The subretinal fluid is sucked out through a puncture in the sclera after the band is in place but before it is tightened.

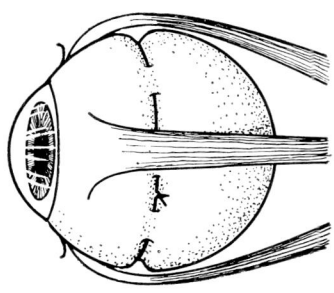

DIAGRAM TO SHOW HOW THE BAND IS PLACED ROUND THE EQUATOR OF THE EYE UNDER THE RECTI MUSCLES AND CONJUNCTIVA IN THE ARRUGA STRING OPERATION FOR RETINAL DETACHMENT

'*Plomb*' operations may be performed where there is a single hole in the retina. A piece of silicone is sutured on to the sclera to produce a localised indentation of the eyeball in contrast to the encircling band.

Whatever operation is done success cannot be promised. The prognosis depends on many factors including the length of time the detachment has been present, on the condition of the retina, on the degree of myopia, and on whether 'holes' in the detachment have been located. The patient is told that an operation is advisable, giving the best possibility of restoring the sight, whereas if the detachment remains untreated the retina will become further separated and at a later date there would be much less chance of an operation improving the sight. It is usually desirable to admit the patient immediately.

Pre-operative care

The aim is to allow the detached retina to become flat again; although it will not be re-attached this makes it possible to examine it thoroughly for a hole or holes in the retina, and then the type of operation can be decided upon. The patient may be nursed in bed with his head in such a position that the detached area of retina will be at the lowest part of the eye and so use the force of gravity to

Surgical Nursing

replace the retina. For example, a patient with the lower half of the retina detached will be nursed propped up in a sitting position; if the upper and outer area of the right eye were detached he should lie on his right side with the foot of the bed raised. It will be necessary to keep the pupil very well dilated for examination purposes. Various instruments are used to get a good view of the fundus such as an indirect ophthalmoscope. This allows the operator to use both eyes and thereby obtain a more complete view of the whole area of the retina. At this time very detailed drawings will be made.

This pre-operative period is a considerable strain on the patient both physically and mentally. It is a difficult adjustment for an active person to be suddenly required to lie flat in one position and he may get muscular pain and considerable disturbance of digestion and bowel activity. He will probably find it difficult to sleep without his usual freedom to turn over. The complete immobility may be a predisposing cause of hypostatic pneumonia or venous thrombosis. Some surgeons do not 'position' their patients pre-operatively, and some will allow a patient who is lying flat to sit up at mealtimes and for toilet purposes. The mental strain is nearly always a problem; the circumstances of sudden admission to hospital with its attendant home complications or difficulties over work, combined with the uncertainty as to the outcome of the sudden loss of sight make the pre-operative days very difficult to get through. The enforced idleness adds to the problem. The physical symptoms are relieved with appropriate treatment and deep-breathing exercises, and gentle leg movements are encouraged as part of the nursing routine. The method of moving the patient will depend on his position in bed, the aim being to alter the position of his head as little as possible. The care of women's hair presents a problem as it is difficult to keep it well combed without undue movement of the head, and the unexpected admission will not have been allowed a wash beforehand. Constipation is best treated with suppositories, and a urinary output chart is useful as a check that enough fluid is being taken. The mental strain may not be apparent in a reserved patient but it is often all the more serious for not being expressed. Medical social workers can help to solve the social problems; visitors may be very helpful and they should be given opportunities to discuss their problems with the hospital staff so as to minimize the

Surgical Nursing

anxiety and responsibility for the patient. The nurses will be in a difficult position in that they cannot reassure the patient or relatives as to the outcome of the operation, and the doctors will not be able to foretell the result, but a sympathetic attitude to the particular problem is always appreciated. The patient is usually helped by sedative drugs and he is probably happier in a ward with other patients rather than in a single room. Whichever operation is chosen the local preparation will include cutting the eye-lashes and cleansing the lids. The pupil must be fully dilated to allow fundus examination, and for the same reason the cornea must be kept perfectly clear—if cocaine drops are used and the eye allowed to remain open the corneal surface becomes dry and slightly hazy.

Post-operative care

The time for which it is considered necessary to immobilize the patient after operation is shorter now. It used to be thought that the retina would remain reattached following operation if the eye could be kept as still as possible for two to three weeks. To this end both eyes were bandaged and the pre-operative procedure of positioning the patient in relation to the hole in the retina was continued. The more recent opinion is that complete immobilization is not of great importance and some surgeons will cover one eye only. The day on which the patient is allowed to get up will depend on the site of the operation; for instance if it is in the lower part of the eye, the patient will be allowed up sooner than if the site is above. The variation in treatment makes it difficult for older nurses to adjust their ideas but they will welcome the lessening of the strain on the patient of the long post-operative period in bed.

The care of the eyes. The dressing is usually changed on the second or third day and then daily unless there is special indication for more frequent treatment. If both eyes are covered, the Moorfield's Bandage (see p. 111) allows the dressing to be done without any movement of the head. It may be helpful to have the curtains or blind partly drawn as the eyes are very sensitive to light when both have been covered. Atropine is usually ordered and it is important to notice the degree of dilatation of the pupil as the surgeon cannot examine the eye satisfactorily unless the pupil is large. 'Vaseline' gauze or some

Surgical Nursing

lubricant on the eye pads helps to keep them comfortably in place on the eyes.

Conjunctival sutures can be removed on the fourth day but they are often left longer if not causing any discomfort. Patients may then be allowed to wear their own glasses.

When it was considered very important to keep the eye as still as possible, 'pinhole glasses' were ordered for use as soon as the double eye pads were removed. These have a small aperture in the centre of each eyepiece with the object of limiting the movements of the eyes as the patient can only see when looking straight forward. His own spectacles can be made to serve the same purpose if the lenses are covered by dark paper with a three-millimetre hole at the optical centre; dark paper side-pieces can be fixed to the frames. Most surgeons do not now consider this to be necessary and the patient is allowed to wear his own spectacles as soon as the conjunctival sutures have been removed.

When the patient gets up he should be warned of the risk of knocking into things due to the limited field of vision. He must avoid any sudden jar such as that due to slipping in the bath or tripping over a mat. He should avoid any severe exertion until given permission by the surgeon.

If the retina does not remain in place at the first attempt, the surgeon may repeat the operation.

SQUINT

Strabismus (Gr. to turn) or squint is a condition in which the visual axes of the eyes are not parallel to each other. Normally the movements of both eyes are co-ordinated so that the axes are parallel except when the eyes converge for looking at a close object.

Strabismus is called by the colloquial terms 'a cast', 'a lazy eye', or by the phrases 'the eyes are crossed' or 'his eye goes in the corner'.

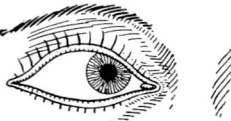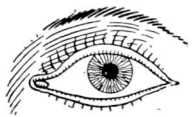

RIGHT CONVERGENT SQUINT

Surgical Nursing

It is more usual for the eye to turn in, a convergent squint, but it may diverge or occasionally turn up or down.

It is usually due to the fact that the eyes are not seeing objects clearly when used together, and to overcome this difficulty one eye is unconsciously turned away from the object. This slightly blurred sight may be due to the need for spectacles, and when the correct ones are worn the squint will be improved or cured.

A squint most often becomes apparent in childhood and is often first noticed after an illness such as measles.

Treatment of Squint

Refraction. Children's eyes are tested under a mydriatic, usually atropine: it is common for atropine ointment to be ordered to *both eyes* for a few days before the test. The mother should be told that this will make the pupils large and the sight blurred for reading, so that the child cannot do close work at school during the time.

If glasses are ordered it is most important that they are worn constantly; many mothers, who can afford it, have two pairs so that if one is broken or bent the child will not be without them.

Spectacles for an Infant. The side pieces end in wire loops instead of curling behind the ears. Tape should be threaded through the loops and tied on top of the head (see p. 180).

Occlusion. The occlusion of one eye may be necessary. The sight in the squinting eye often deteriorates from lack of use and by covering the good eye the child is obliged to use the weaker one with consequent improvement. It is not usually sufficient to cover the spectacle glass as the child can squint round it. Various methods of occlusion are used, the most important part being the lower nasal side for a converging eye. The eye can be covered with Elastoplast. Lint spread with ointment is laid over the closed lids and the eyebrow to prevent adhesion to the hair and lashes. Elastoplast, three-inch width is applied over the eye; special care is needed over the bridge of the nose and down the side of it. This type of occlusion requires good cooperation on the part of the mother; she will naturally dislike having the child's face covered and it is very difficult to keep it reasonably clean. She can be shown how to re-apply fresh Elastoplast and it is

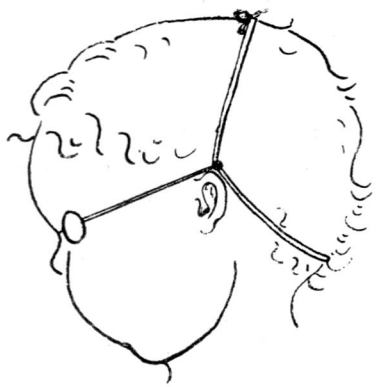

SPECTACLES FOR AN INFANT

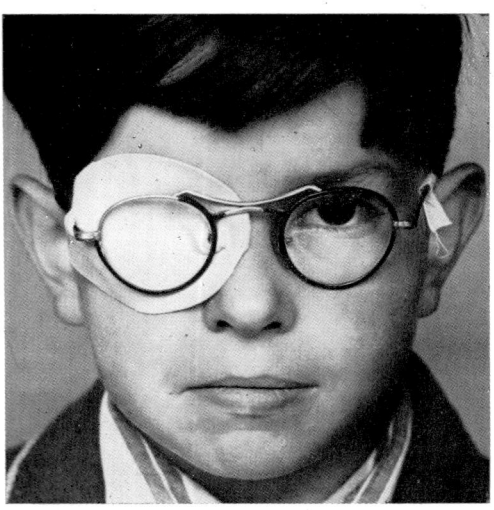

XLVIII. Occlusion applied to the spectacle frame. The Elastoplast is doubled so that no adhesive surface sticks to the skin. *N.B.* As this boy was an in-patient his glasses were marked with his name to prevent the children's glasses getting muddled

Surgical Nursing

often most encouraging to see how well the mothers manage this tiresome treatment (see plate XLVIII).

There are patent occluders, e.g. Doyne's Occluder, made for attachment to the spectacles; they do not fit the face so accurately but are convenient if the occlusion is for certain hours daily. Later it may be adequate to cover part of the spectacle lens with opaque material.

The mother must be warned that the child will dislike not being able to see as clearly as usual and it will probably make him tired and irritable. She must be careful that he does not knock things over or hurt himself, due to the limited sight. Crossing the road in traffic is specially dangerous.

The results of occlusion are often surprisingly satisfactory and well worth the trouble.

Orthoptic Treatment. Orthoptic treatment, or 'squint exercises', are carried out by specially trained orthoptists, by means of various instruments which re-educate the child to use both eyes at once. For satisfactory results they must be done regularly, perhaps two or three times a week for twenty minutes to half an hour. This is a considerable tie to the mother. They are used both before and after operation.

Squint Operations. The operations consist of shortening or lengthening various muscles which move the eyeball.

A muscle can be shortened by 'resection' and 'advancement', a piece of tendon being cut out and the end sewn on to the sclera nearer to the cornea. A muscle can be lengthened by 'tenotomy', the cutting of some fibres of the muscle to weaken its action; in 'recession' the muscle is cut off at its attachment to the sclera, and sewn on further back. The operation is nearly always performed under general anaesthesia.

Post-operative Care. The nursing depends on the type of operation and on the individual surgeon's wishes. Because mothers are now encouraged to be admitted with the child or to visit for much of the day, the experience of undergoing a squint operation is not nearly so traumatic as it used to be. It is usual for young children to be admitted, have the operation and go home in a few days. The eyes are seldom covered after the operation. The child is usually assessed by the Orthoptist on the first post-operative day. She will give instruc-

Surgical Nursing

tions to the nursing staff and to the parents as to whether the child should wear glasses and whether or not he is allowed to do close work or play with toys which require him to converge and accommodate to see them clearly. A child with a convergent squint is usually discouraged from doing close work.

Local Treatment. The eyes are apt to discharge slightly and the parents should be instructed to swab them gently twice daily; antibiotic drops may be ordered.

Observations to be made after squint operations.

1. The presence of any discharge.

2. Whether the stitches are in place: the conjunctival ones sometimes fall out.

3. The operative result. This is assessed by standing in front of the child and getting him to look straight ahead at a distant object. The corneal reflex is used as a guide to the position of the eyes. If the patient is facing a window or an artificial light, the light reflex will show on both corneae and if the eyes are straight, the reflex will be in the same place on both eyes: if one eye is converging, the reflex will appear to be further out compared with that on the other eye and, conversely, if the eye is diverging the reflex will be nearer to the nasal side of one cornea. Nurses will need some practice

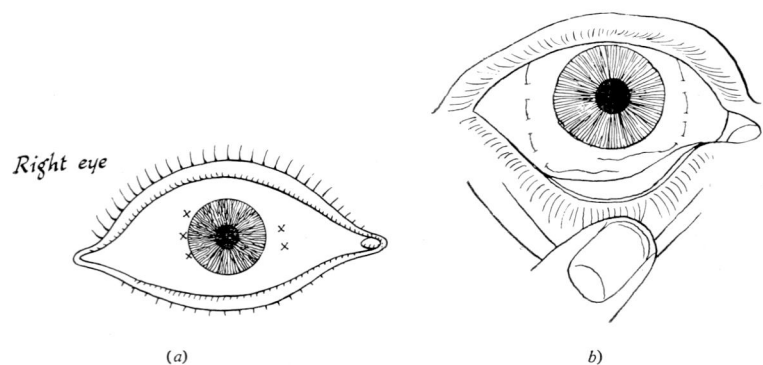

(*a*) Interrupted sutures.

(*b*) Continuous 'running' sutures through conjunctiva only.

SQUINT OPERATION SUTURES

Surgical Nursing

in making these observations. If the child wears glasses these will reduce the angle of the squint and should be worn when assessing the result of the operation.

Conjunctival Sutures. These may be of black silk or catgut. Interrupted black silk sutures will fall out of their own accord, but running sutures must be removed and the child will return to hospital on about the fifth post-operative day for this to be carried out. Catgut sutures will be absorbed. Conjunctival sutures can be removed after a few days but in some cases the suture passes through muscle as well as conjunctiva and must not be removed without the surgeon's instructions as the length of time may depend on the operative results. *See p. 87 for details of the removal of sutures.*

The results of operations for squint cannot be guaranteed as immediately successful: they have often to be followed by orthoptic treatment, sometimes by further operation and frequently by the constant use of spectacles. For this reason it is very important that the parents should have an opportunity to discuss it with the surgeon before consent is given.

Young adults often desire an operation for squint for cosmetic reasons: in some cases this is highly successful, but it is not always possible owing to a troublesome diplopia when the eyes are straight.

The following leaflet is used in one ophthalmic hospital and is often given to parents by a surgeon after he has spoken to them about their child.

"Squints in Children

The following notes have been written so that you may understand and help in the treatment, if you have a child who squints.

Squinting means being cross-eyed: that is, the two eyes look in different directions. Usually one eye turns in; occasionally one eye may turn out.

Squinting does *not* mean 'screwing the eyes up' or peering.

Most cases can be cured, but it is important to begin treatment early, as soon as the squint is noticed, because the longer a squint has lasted, the more difficult it becomes to cure, and after a time it becomes impossible to cure. A child should never be left 'to grow out of it' as that seldom, if ever, happens, and if the eye does become straight again, it usually becomes a 'lazy eye', that is an eye with very defective sight.

It is important to realize that treatment will probably extend over a long period. Many cases require spectacles as part of the treatment.

If the sight in the squinting eye is poor, it may be necessary to cover up the good eye in order to make the poorer eye work and improve its sight. This covering up must be done effectively and thoroughly and you will be shown how to do it. If after a time it is found that the originally good (or covered) eye now turns in while the other remains straight, this is *not* a cause for alarm but is a good sign as it means that the sight of the old squinting eye has improved. The eye specialist will tell you how to proceed. No eye should be covered for more than one month without the child seeing the specialist, or orthoptist.

If the sight in both eyes is fairly good or if and when the weaker eye had improved sufficiently, *some* cases are helped by special exercises, and this treatment may be advised for your child. (The exercises are carried out at special clinics by specially qualified experts, and usually necessitate one or two weekly treatments for many weeks.) *Not* all cases are suitable or benefited by exercises, but if they are likely to help your child, you will be told. An operation may be necessary in addition to other treatment, and glasses may still have to be worn afterwards.

Lastly, it may be desirable to operate to improve the appearance of the child."

ENUCLEATION OF AN EYE

Reasons for the operation. Excision of the eyeball is only undertaken for a *blind eye which is painful* or for an eye which is a danger to the patient's health. The common reason is pain in a blind eye, but a surgeon will seldom advise the operation until the pain is sufficiently severe to make the patient ask the surgeon to do it. There are a few rare *malignant growths* of eye, e.g. retinoblastoma, for which excision is necessary to prevent metastases; unfortunately these sometimes occur in infants. The condition of *sympathetic ophthalmia* is one in which the damaged eye causes acute inflammation in the second eye,

Surgical Nursing

endangering the sight of that also: if it is recognized early, removal of the damaged eye will be advised.

The operation is a comparatively minor one, but the fact of losing an eye is always a serious shock to the patient. When obtaining the signed consent to operation, it is important that the patient or his parents are absolutely clear as to what is involved and the words 'removal of right (or left) eye' on the written form, may be preferable to 'enucleation' or 'excision of eye'. The same applies to the explanation through an interpreter in a foreign language when there is some risk that it is not clearly understood especially if the interpreter thinks it is kinder not to shock the patient. If a child is old enough to understand, it is usually wiser to tell him before the operation; a child respects and trusts people who do not deceive him and it could be a terrible shock to find out later that it had been done without his knowledge. It is necessary to have a form of consent signed by the patient, or by the parents in the case of a minor.

Pre-operative Treatment. The eye-lashes are sometimes cut as it makes it easier to keep the lids clean after operation.

In some hospitals it is the practice to mark the forehead of the side for operation with a small piece of adhesive strapping before the patient leaves the ward to prevent the remote possibility of the wrong eye being removed.

It is usual to give the patient a general anaesthetic, but the operation may be performed under a local anaesthetic if the patient is in poor general health.

Post-operative Treatment. After operation a firm pad is bandaged over the lids to prevent the formation of a haematoma of the socket: the pressure bandage should not be loosened until the next day. In the usual operation, the conjunctiva is sutured, but some surgeons stitch a small plastic or light metal globe inside it with the aim of improving the movement of the artificial eye. In the latter case no pressure bandage is applied and the patient may be kept in bed for a few days until the tissues have healed over it. If there is no globe in the socket, the patient is allowed to get up as soon as his general condition will permit.

Local Treatment. The socket often discharges a little and will require swabbing or irrigation twice a day.

Surgical Nursing

The conjunctival stitches are removed on about the fifth day and the pad and bandage can be replaced by opaque paper covering the spectacle glass or an eye shade.

Artificial Eye. This cannot be fitted until the socket has settled for a few weeks. A plastic shell is worn after the first few days and that is then replaced by an artificial eye made specially for the patient.

Other Operations for the Removal of an Eye

Evisceration. In this operation the cornea and the contents of the eyeball are removed, leaving the sclera. The method prevents the necessity of cutting through the optic nerve which is of advantage in acute infection of the eye. The after-care is the same as for excision, bearing in mind that the patient may have been more acutely ill beforehand.

Exenteration of Orbit. In this operation the lids and the tissues within the orbit are removed with the eye. It is performed for malignant conditions such as rodent ulcer of lid. The cavity will require dressing and plugging, and there may be subsequent plastic operations to reproduce lids. A prosthesis representing eyelids and eye can be fitted to a spectacle frame with a very good cosmetic result.

Artificial Eyes

Artificial eyes are made to resemble the front of the eye and are shell-shaped, being hollow behind. Patients are usually advised to remove it at night, as they would dentures, but the modern preference is for the prosthesis to be left undisturbed unless there is discharge from the socket. The artificial eye must be carefully washed and kept in a box or container as it is an expensive and precious article: the work of making them is highly skilled and each patient

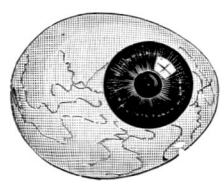

ARTIFICIAL EYE

Surgical Nursing

has his eye specially matched and made. The older type are breakable and the edges tend to get rough after about a year's wear; most of the recent ones are of plastic material. Patients who are particular about their appearance may have one with a slightly larger pupil for use in the evening in less bright light.

Method of Removing an Artificial Eye

The patient learns to do this very skilfully for himself, but the nurse must be prepared to do it when necessary. A glass rod or special instrument is required. The patient should be lying down if the nurse is inexperienced, as it is very easy for the eye to slip from the fingers and fall on the floor, whereas if the head is on a pillow the eye will come to no harm. The patient is asked to look up, the lower lid is drawn down and the glass rod is passed under the lower edge of the eye which is then lifted over the lower lid. With slight pressure through the upper lid the eye is pressed out of the socket,

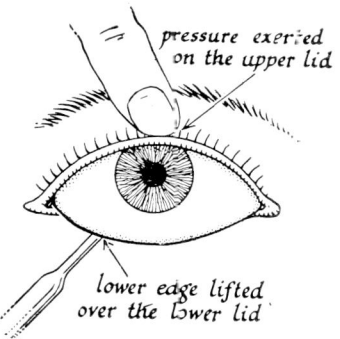

REMOVAL OF ARTIFICIAL EYE

care being taken to hold it securely as it is removed. This is usually quite simple, but it can be a little difficult in a young person with a strong orbicularis muscle of the lid, or in an older patient with a very deep socket.

To Replace an Artificial Eye

The upper side is known by a shallow notch towards the nasal end which is made for the pulley of the superior oblique muscle. The

Surgical Nursing

eye slips in more easily if it is wet. The upper lid is raised and the pointed nasal end of the eye is slipped under the lid; the eye is then rotated to its correct position, the lower lid is drawn down and the lower side allowed to slip into the lower fornix.

Research is being undertaken on implants for sockets with the aim of giving better movement to the artificial eye; there are various patterns made of plastic materials and the rectus muscles are sutured to them; in these cases the prosthesis may have a prong or hole or magnet incorporated in it, to hold it in position on the implant. The insertion and removal of the prosthesis has to be done with a special rubber sucker similar to that used for removing contact lenses. The present disadvantage of these implants is that the sockets tend to become irritated and inflamed but this is thought to be due to the materials used and it is hoped that research will result in ones that can be retained satisfactorily.

OPERATIONS ON THE LACHRYMAL PASSAGES

Disease of the lachrymal passages often results in an obstruction to the drainage of excess tears which normally pass through the tear ducts to the back of the nose. It will be remembered that when starting to cry one sniffs and wants to blow one's nose, before the tears spill over the eyelid and trickle down the cheek. It is like rain which will normally collect in gutters and run into the drains leaving the road dry, but in a very heavy thunderstorm the drains cannot take the amount of rain water and they overflow. The obstruction may be in the lower canaliculus or in the naso-lachrymal duct, and can be investigated by syringing fluid through the passages (see page 83). Occasionally the obstruction may be due to abnormalities in the nose. If the naso-lachrymal duct is the site of obstruction the sac will remain filled with tears and the fluid may become infected owing to the lack of drainage; sometimes an abscess forms and if it bursts through the skin it may leave a discharging sinus. Infection of the sac is *dacryocystitis*, and the rare condition of infection of the lachrymal gland is *dacryoadenitis*.

When the excess tears cannot drain away the patient complains of a watering eye; epiphora is the term used when watering is due to

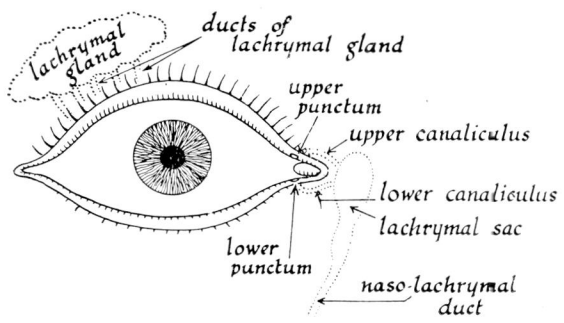

LACHRYMAL APPARATUS

defective drainage, whereas lacrimation describes excessive secretion of tears. Epiphora is an annoying condition which is more troublesome in cold and windy weather; when there is no blockage of the lachrymal channels it can be due to displacement of the lower punctum caused by ectropion, which is an eversion of the lower lid resulting in the punctum being drawn away from the eyeball.

Operations on the Lachrymal Passages
Probing

The particular use of lachrymal probing is for the obstruction which occurs in infants; this is a condition which is present at birth due to incomplete canalization of the naso-lachrymal duct. It shows as slight discharge in the nasal corner of the eye which is otherwise healthy. The treatment consists of digital pressure over the sac to express any secretion which collects in it and the mother is taught to do this at each feeding time and then to wipe away the discharge and instil antibiotic drops (see page 80). If there is no improvement the surgeon may pass a probe under general anaesthesia when the baby is several months old, and this nearly always results in a complete cure.

Operations for Obstruction of the Lower Canaliculus

Obstruction may result from different causes which include infection of some duration, injury involving the nasal end of the lower lid,

Surgical Nursing

and irradiation for the treatment of a rodent ulcer in that region. Owing to the very narrow lumen of the canaliculus there is difficulty in maintaining the patency made by operation. It is usual for a length of polythene tubing to be left in position for several weeks or months; this is sometimes uncomfortable and annoying cosmetically but if it can be tolerated it provides the best hope of a cure.

Operations for Obstruction of the Naso-Lachrymal Duct

This site of obstruction is the most common and the condition seems to occur without apparent cause in middle or old age, women being more frequently affected than men. If the condition is treated soon after the onset of the watering eye, syringing at intervals of several days may overcome the obstruction. Before deciding to operate, the surgeon usually requires a dacryocystogram X-ray, an opaque solution being introduced to show the site of the blockage. If there is any history of nasal trouble a specialist's opinion will be obtained. The operation of choice is a *dacryocystorhinostomy*, which involves making an opening from the lachrymal sac directly into the nasal cavity, and in this way by-passing the naso-lachrymal duct. In some cases a length of polythene tubing is left in position and this will eventually be removed from the nostril. The skin incision will be in the line of the fold of skin at the side of the nose and leaves almost no scar. After-treatment will include gentle sac syringing until patency is assured.

Excision of Lachrymal Sac

This is occasionally performed when circumstances make it desirable to avoid a longer operation, or when there has been gross infection in the sac. This operation will not cure the watering of the eye but it will prevent recurrent infection of the sac, and it might be of value in reducing the risk of infection before cataract operation in a very old person.

PLASTIC OPERATIONS TO LIDS

These may be performed for a number of conditions, e.g. ectropion, entropion, rodent ulcer, ptosis, injuries, etc.

The post-operative nursing aims at:

Surgical Nursing

1. Keeping the area clean. 2. If a skin graft has been applied, keeping it in position by good bandaging. 3. Keeping the cornea healthy. In certain cases stitches might irritate it or in others there may be slight exposure as after the correction of ptosis. 4. Sutures should only be removed at the surgeon's request as it is not always apparent if they are superficial or if they are through muscle or fascia. If they are deep in the lower fornix it may be necessary to have an assistant who is experienced in holding the lid in the required position.

These patients often have their operations as Day Cases but they may require admission for a few days.

10

NOTES ON OPHTHALMIC THEATRE WORK

A special ophthalmic theatre is usually provided owing to the nature of work. The particular requirements are:

Quiet. The surgeon is operating within a very limited field and any sudden noise must be avoided especially during lens extractions when the incision is being made and when the lens is being delivered.

In Eye Hospitals the theatre may have several small operating rooms with central sterilizing arrangements.

Good lighting and arrangements to darken the theatre. Daylight is ideal for general preparations and if possible there should be one large window facing north. The blind should be such that it can be rapidly drawn down to darken the room completely: several operations require a dark theatre or ophthalmoscopic examination may be necessary during the procedures.

SPECIAL EQUIPMENT

Illumination. In addition to an overhead operating lamp there may be a special lamp which gives shadowless illumination.

Operating Microscope. Many surgeons now use an operating microscope. This is of great assistance in very delicate operations where small instruments and very fine sutures are being used.

Instrument Sterilizers. The use of boiling sterilizers is now discouraged but if it is necessary to use one it should be large enough to take a special tray with a perforated bottom; the tray is lifted out with the instruments in it, thus saving further handling in setting them

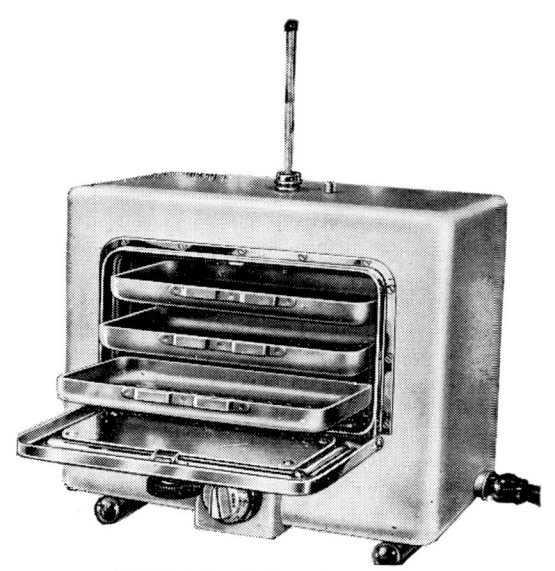

XLIX. Electric hot air sterilizer

separately on the trolley. The sterilizer is filled with distilled water to prevent furring of the instruments.

Dry Sterilization. Dry heat is ideal for the sterilization of ophthalmic instruments. Modern theatres are equipped with electric ovens which are thermostatically controlled (see plate XLIX). For each operation the set of instruments, including sutures, is arranged on a rack in a tray with a well-fitting lid (see p. 194); the tray is wrapped in stout brown paper and sterilized in the oven for an hour at a temperature of 160° C. When required for use, the tray is set on the instrument trolley and at the beginning of the operation the flat lid can be placed beside the tray so that used instruments are put into it. It has been found that the blades of knives are harmed by a temperature above 150° C and therefore they must be sterilized separately and are often put into glass tubes. The knife is clipped into a small rack for protection and the end of the glass tube is sealed with a special cap (see p. 194). The end of the tube can be covered with Cellophane and adhesive tape or it can be closed by a short tube of slightly wider diameter which is put over the open end and secured with adhesive tape. The advantages

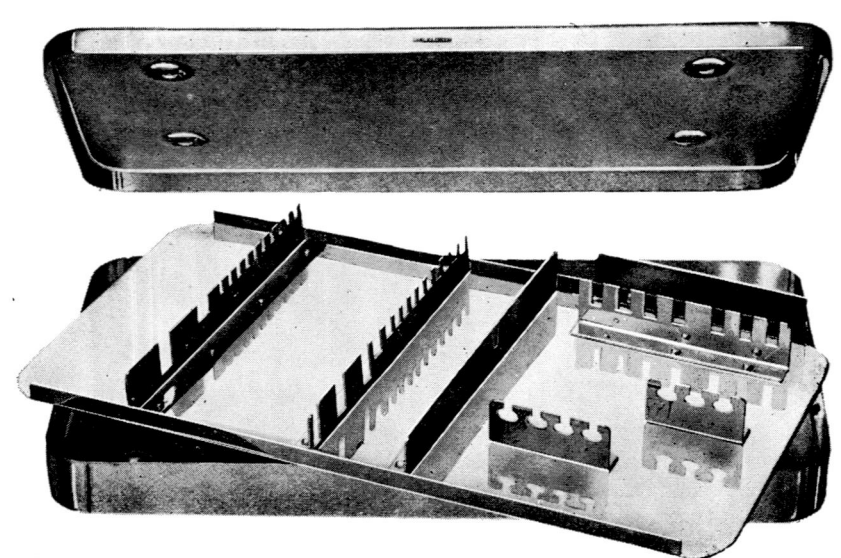

L. Sterilizer box

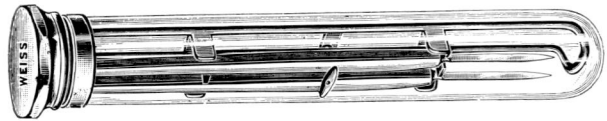

KNIFE RACK IN TUBE

of dry sterilization are that there is no reliance on antiseptic solutions for knives and they are not rinsed or handled in any way after being selected. Also an emergency set of instruments can be kept in readiness. The disadvantage is the length of time required for sterilization which makes it necessary to have sufficient instruments to prepare all the trays for cases to be done in one operating session. For this reason the theatre may also have an alternative water sterilizer so that additional instruments can be prepared at short notice.

Instrument Trolleys. These are smaller than for general use. Square ones 18 inches by 18 inches, are convenient, and there should be

Notes on Ophthalmic Theatre Work

sufficient to allow several to be laid up at one time. In some theatres the instruments are set on stands which can be swung across the patient's chest.

Magnets. Giant and hand magnets are required for the removal of intra-ocular foreign bodies. There are many patterns of electromagnets. The theatre staff should be careful to remove their watches before a large magnet is switched on (see Plates LI and LII).

Diathermy Machine. The use of diathermy for retinal detachment has largely been replaced by cryo therapy.

Cryo Machine. This machine is used mainly for cryo therapy for retinal detachment and for cryo extraction of lens. The machine has on it a cylinder of gas, usually carbon dioxide, and has special cryo probes connected to it. When the machine is switched on the gas will be released and the tip of the probe will freeze.

THEATRE TECHNIQUE

The best preparation for ophthalmic work is a period of training in a first-class general theatre. The nurse who has sound general experience can adapt the principles to eye work where the less rigid technique may confuse the inexperienced. At the present time some surgeons do not wear rubber gloves and will 'wash up' for a shorter length of time than five minutes; they argue that they never handle the tissues with their fingers and that results prove that their technique is satisfactory.

If instruments and bowls are not dry sterilized, they should be boiled according to the rules of the particular hospital; three minutes is usually considered to be sufficient.

Antiseptics or dry heat are used for the sterilization of sharp instruments as even the most careful boiling will harm the delicate edge. Hospitals have their own sterilizing solutions, but care must be taken that ivory handles are not put into one containing Lysol.

The theatre sister's work will vary according to the practice of individual surgeons and the size of the operating unit. Most surgeons require a sister or nurse to be 'scrubbed up' to attend to the instrument trolley; where there is not an experienced House Surgeon some rely on the sister to assist with the operations, whereas a few prefer to take their own instruments and threaded sutures off a prepared

LI. Philps Giant eye magnet

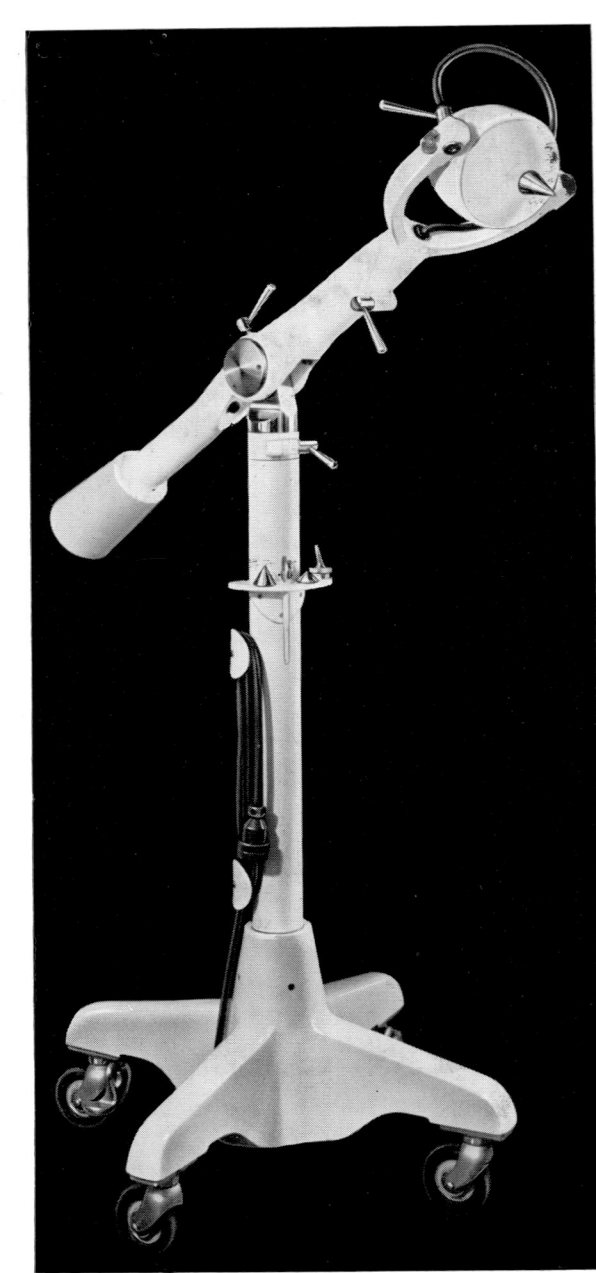

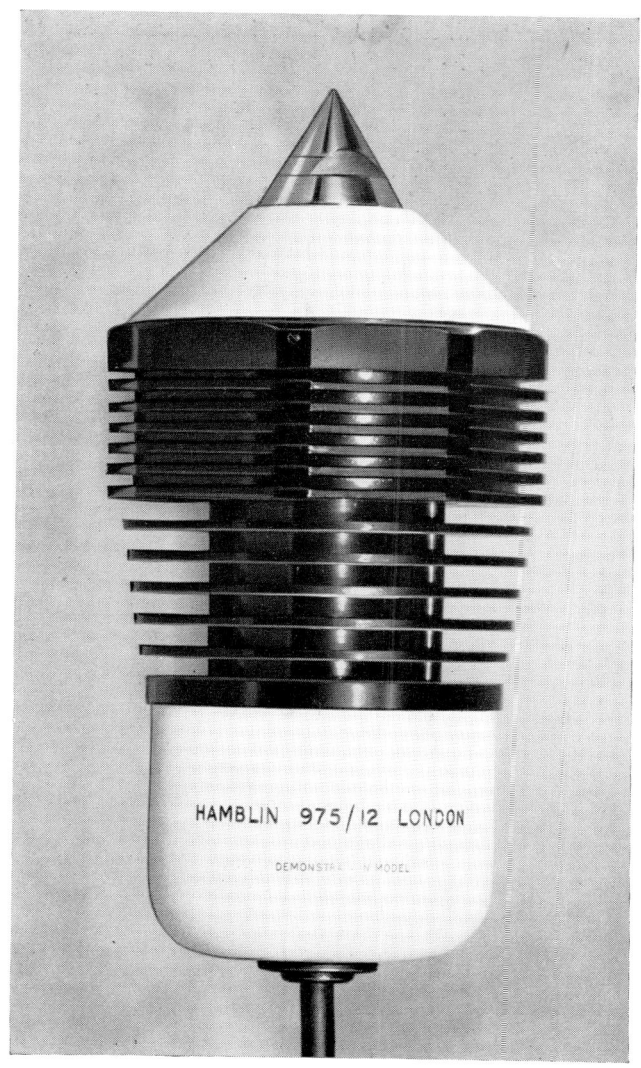

LII. Portable magnet

This portable magnet has a variety of points which are detachable for sterilization. Although it is only 5½ inches in length the magnet is very heavy and the surgeon would use it held in both hands

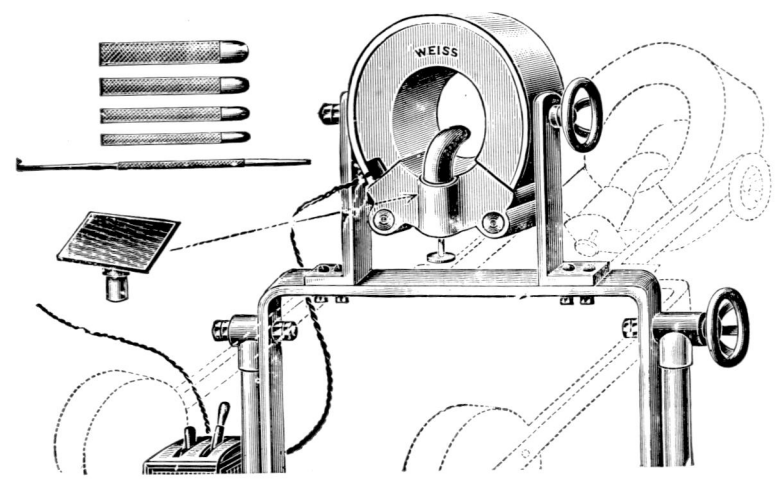

MELLINGER'S RING MAGNET

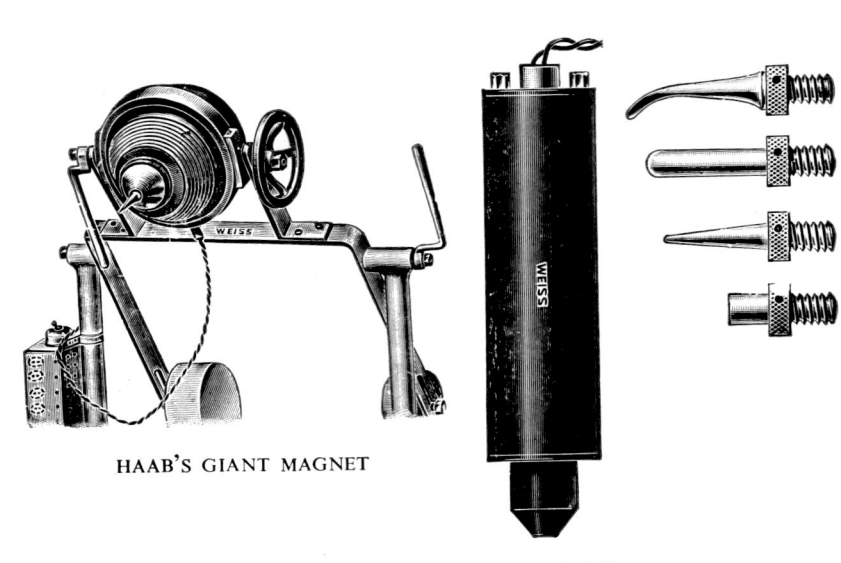

HAAB'S GIANT MAGNET

HAND MAGNET

Notes on Ophthalmic Theatre Work

trolley. Even if the surgeons do not wear gloves for all operations, the sister may find it better and quicker if she wears them for her work as the time between cases is often brief.

Care of Instruments. In a book of this scope it is not possible to illustrate complete lists of instruments for each operation, but the theatre sister must keep an up-to-date log-book giving the requirements for every operation with the special variations for different surgeons; a good-quality loose-leaf book is useful for the purpose so that alterations and additions can easily be made. An ophthalmic instrument catalogue is invaluable when ordering or sending instruments for repair and is good for teaching student nurses.

An accurate instrument inventory is most necessary owing to the fact that instruments have to be sent to special instrument makers for sharpening and they are often away for many weeks. A new nurse will be surprised at the numbers of each variety of knife until she realizes how frequently they require sharpening.

Knives. These are kept in velvet-lined boxes and if not in regular use the blades should be smeared with a very little lubricant. The cutting edge can be very easily spoilt and a theatre sister is well advised to handle them entirely herself. They should be lifted out of the box by depressing the end of the handle so that there is no chance of the point being pressed downwards.

The use of each instrument must be known for the intelligent handling of it: for example, that the whole length of the blade of a cataract knife is used in a sawing movement, or that one of a pair of twin knives has a blunt end. Repeated sharpening will render some too short for their original purpose, but they can be reserved for other uses.

Testing of Knives. The blade should be examined for marks or stains which roughen the surface. The edge and point can be looked at with a corneal loupe and are tested on a Trial Drum. The fine white kid is of about the same texture as cornea and the cutting edge is judged accordingly. The knife should be held so that its own weight will cause it to cut through the kid (see p. 200).

Each knife should be tested immediately before use and again before it is put away in the box. It requires experience to judge when a knife requires sharpening and some surgeons prefer to select their

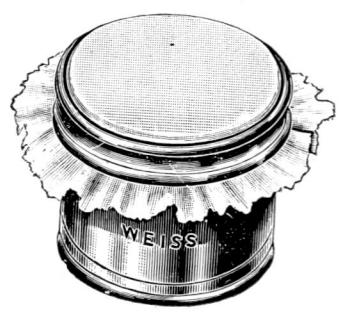

TRIAL DRUM

own before operating. It is a convenient system for storing knives if the new and recently sharpened ones are always put at the back of the boxes. Knives should be placed in a Knife Rack when in sterilizing solution or on a trolley. The cutting edge should be downwards so that a covering towel will not rest upon it. Knives should be dried on fine linen or cambric and be returned immediately to their boxes. De Wecker's Iris Scissors are treated like knives, but other scissors may be sterilized with the instruments.

Trephines need to be carefully dried inside: this is done with a long darning needle threaded with several thicknesses of cotton.

Corneal grafting trephines require special care. They vary in size from 4 mm to 10·1 mm. Some surgeons use a slightly larger one for the patient's eye than that with which they cut the graft and there-

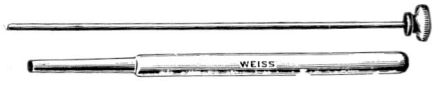

TREPHINE

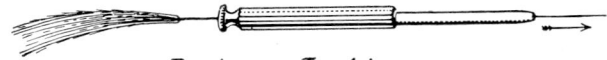

Drying a Trephine

THREADING COTTON THROUGH A TREPHINE

Notes on Ophthalmic Theatre Work

for the Franceschetti trephines are made in pairs, e.g. 4 mm and 4·1 mm, and 5 mm and 5·1 mm, etc. The trephines may not be boiled or put into disinfectant solutions but must be sterilized in a hot-air oven at a temperature of 140° C for one hour. After use the trephine should be wiped dry of aqueous fluid. The obturator should be screwed back to partly withdraw it—it will not come right out without taking the trephine to pieces and that should not be done frequently. The lumen of the trephine will be damp with aqueous and it must be dried without damaging the cutting edge. One way of drying it is with a match on to which are twisted wisps of wool. The trephines should be tested and sent for resharpening as often as necessary.

Other Instruments. It needs a little experience to appreciate the delicacy of the various forceps: iris forceps are specially liable to be pressed apart so that their points do not meet accurately. Metal or plastic rings on the forceps keep their points in position.

Rules for care after use:

1. They must never be collected from the trolley in handfuls as they can so easily be bent.

2. A large bowl of cold water and a toothbrush are used for brushing them after use. There are special solutions available which will dissolve blood and mucus.

3. Should it be necessary to boil instruments they should never be put into the sterilizer until the water is boiling, and it will be possible to dry them immediately they are removed. The routine use of a three-minute egg-timer on the sterilizer lid helps to prevent boiling for too long.

4. They should be dried on a fine towel and laid in an orderly manner on a clean towel.

5. As each pair of forceps is put away the points should be pressed together to see that they meet exactly.

The stainless steel instruments seldom require cleaning if they are dried hot: it is a mistake to polish them unnecessarily as some bending is very liable to occur as the powder is rubbed off. Distilled water in the sterilizer prevents fur collecting on them.

Sutures. Atraumatic sutures are used for most purposes and may be of silk or of man-made fibres such as Dexon. The needles and

Notes on Ophthalmic Theatre Work

suture material will vary with the type of tissue for which they are used. Corneal needles and sutures need to be specially fine, and there are others suitable for muscle, conjunctiva and skin. Atraumatic sutures have the great advantage of reliable sterility and availability as required but, for economy, some sutures are prepared by theatre staff. The most usual material is black and white silk. For instance, sets of sutures for lids usually consist of 3 No. 0 black silk and 1 No. 1 white silk on No. 4 Eye Curved needles. These are threaded on a piece of firm cotton material and are then pre-packed and sterilized in a Hot Air Oven at 145° C for one and a half hours.

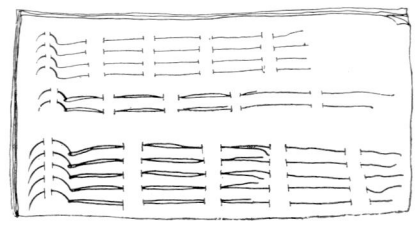

SUTURES THREADED ON FOLDED MUSLIN

Needles. Curved Eye Needles, size 4 or Maddox, are the most commonly used. Between use they can be put into small pieces of chamois leather or pieces of lint which have been spread with a simple ointment. They are easily mislaid during operations and should be counted when the trolley is cleared, as they may be in the used towels. They have to be discarded frequently, being bent or blunt.

The needles tend to become magnetic and difficult to handle and this is specially the case after the instruments have been used with the electromagnet. The magnetism can be removed by using a watch maker's demagnetizing coil.

It is advisable to take new needles for thick silk sutures as these are used when the needle must be put through the tough sclera in a squint operation.

Lotions. For anterior chamber washouts it is strongly advised that all lotions should be supplied in sterile ampoules.

Notes on Ophthalmic Theatre Work

The Care of the Patient in the Theatre. Occasionally patients may be unfit for general anaesthesia, in which case they are bound to be apprehensive and a little conversation helps them very much besides allowing the nurse to observe if they are particularly nervous, deaf, etc. Any relevant information should be passed on to the surgeon before he starts to operate.

Patients often ask if the operation will be painful. It is impossible to know what they feel during operations, but experience shows that very few of them complain that it is painful. It is certainly a mental strain, but most eye operations are very quick—a cataract operation only takes a short time once the preparations are completed. The nurse can assure the patient that the eye will be made quite insensitive and he should feel very little; if he does, he should tell the surgeon who will give him more local anaesthetic.

The time of waiting in the anaesthetic room adds considerably to the patient's apprehension: with good teamwork among all the staff the theatre sister can reduce this to a minimum, but it is one of her problems owing to the short time the cases take.

The older patients may be uncomfortable on the theatre table, and there should be a spare pillow and blanket for use as required.

The theatre nurse must look at the patient's notes and immediately put in anaesthetic drops; this will allow time for extra ones should the eye require them. The eyes ought to be kept closed between instillations.

If it is an intra-ocular operation the nurse is responsible for looking at the result of the culture and reporting if it is not there or if the result is doubtful.

The lashes are usually cut in the ward but this can be done after the patient has been anaesthetised: this is always so in the case of a child.

According to the theatre arrangements the nurse may be responsible for the skin preparation, irrigation and the putting on of the towels.

While the surgeon is operating, the theatre should be completely quiet and the nurses should move about as little as possible. Opening doors, running taps and whispered conversations are all disturbing but particularly so during an intra-ocular operation.

Notes on Ophthalmic Theatre Work

Ophthalmic theatre work gains in human interest from the fact that the patients are not always anaesthetized. A second advantage is that a nurse can see the details of each operation which adds considerably to her understanding of the special nursing required.

APPENDICES

I

EYE DRESSINGS AND SPECIAL EQUIPMENT

EYE SWABS

There are many varieties of swabs favoured by the different ophthalmic hospitals. Whatever material is used for swabs it should be soft and absorbent. The swabs must be prepared in conveniently small pieces so that there is no temptation to excessive economy.

White Lint Swabs

Method of folding line from a twelve-inch roll.

For the cutting of it strong and sharp scissors are essential.

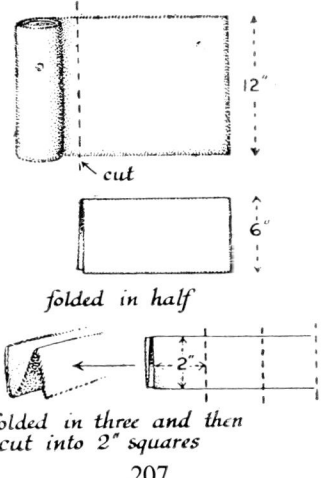

cut

folded in half

folded in three and then cut into 2" squares

Eye Dressings

The size of the swab is important as it must be large enough to protect the fingers from contamination: the tendency is for the swabs to be cut too small. A two-inch square is satisfactory: to ensure that the correct size is maintained the folding of the lint should be done in a certain way.

Eye Swabs

Special gauze and wool swabs are available and consist of a very thin layer of wool between fine gauze; this has the advantage of absorbency without the fluffiness of wool.

In a general ward where there are no special eye swabs white wool can be used either in the form of prepared wool balls or by breaking a piece of autoclaved wool into small pieces. Some eye units use wool swabs in preference to lint ones.

Disposable Tissues

Disposable tissues are very useful for clinic work which involves the instillation of drops. Boxes of tissues $8\frac{3}{4}$ inches by 5 inches are a convenient and economical size and the boxes can be put into dispensing holders fixed to a wall (see p. 47).

Swab Sticks

If swab sticks are not supplied ready prepared, orange sticks should be cut into three-inch lengths and then wisps of white wool are applied to one end. The swab sticks should be autoclaved and are usually moistened before use.

Swabs for Theatre Use

Gauze swabs two-inch square and four-inch square are most generally used, but finer material is necessary for intra-ocular operations or where the cornea must be touched. Soft gauze is used and the swabs may be obtained ready-made or they can be prepared by hand. In the latter case they are made from 1-inch Ribbon Gauze: they must be stitched so that the raw edges are hidden.

Spontex is a synthetic sponge material which is supplied in sheets or strips. It is cut into small cubes and used damp. For sterilization it can be autoclaved and damped with sterile saline prior to use.

Eye Dressings

EYE PADS

The special eye pads are made of white wool between layers of very fine gauze. They are manufactured as single and double pads. If pads are to be improvised care must be taken that wool is never against the eye, owing to the risk of tiny particles getting between the lids and irritating the cornea. Good quality gamgee may be cut to the required shape, but the covering gauze is not so soft as that on the special pads.

The single pads are oval approximately 3 inches long by $2\frac{1}{2}$ inches wide and they cover the eye and rest on the bony orbital ridge; in this way they do not press on the eye. If it is desirable to keep the lids firmly closed a smaller pad can be improvised which fits inside the orbital margin and if it is strapped firmly in place, it will prevent the lid from partly opening with each movement of the other eye.

INDIVIDUAL PACKS OF DRESSINGS AND INSTRUMENTS

The new method of preparing dressings in individual packs is an advance on our older way of using drums from which dressings are taken with Cheatle's forceps. The special paper bags which are self-sealing can be filled with swabs and pads according to the requirements of each hospital, allowing a pack for every treatment. Similarly instruments and sets of equipment which are dry sterilized in advance provide better aseptic conditions for casualty and ward work. The following is a list of sets of instruments which are commonly used in casualty and out-patient departments.

SUGGESTED CONTENTS OF STERILIZED PACKS

For suturing lids and conjunctiva
- 1 Needleholder
- 1 pair Iris Scissors
- 1 pair Lister's suture and conjunctival forceps
- 1 pair Suture forceps
- 2 Atraumatic sutures, black silk, 5–0
- 1 pair forceps for taking Vaseline Petroleum Jelly gauze

Eye Dressings

1 towel clip
1 gallipot for Cetavlon
12 gauze swabs 2 inches by 2 inches
12 swab sticks
2 towels
1 eye pad
(1 guarded speculum in an individual pack)

For removal of corneal foreign body
1 Saunder's needle or other foreign body instrument in a tube
8 swabs
4 swab sticks
1 eye pad
(1 dental burr in a separate pack)

For carbolizing or iodizing a corneal ulcer
1 speculum with lash guards
3 triangular pieces of filter paper
2 sharpened match sticks
1 pannikin or other very small container for carbolic
8 swabs
1 eye pad

For epilation of lashes
1 pair epilation forceps
6 swabs

For incision and curettage of Meibomian cyst
1 No. 3 Bard Parker holder with 'E' blade
1 Meibomian clamp
1 set of 3 Meibomian curettes
1 gallipot for Cetavlon
12 swabs
6 swab sticks
1 lint flap
2 towels
(1 pair Iris scissors and 1 pair Conjunctival forceps in a separate pack)

Eye Dressings

For syringing lacrimal sac
  1 luerlock 2 ml syringe and
  1 luerfitting sac cannula *or*   1 disposable 2 ml syringe and ⎫
                                   1 record fitting sac cannula ⎭

  1 punctum dilator
  1 small container for saline
  6 swabs
   (in separate packs:
   (a) very fine sac cannula
   (b) set of lacrimal probes
   (c) punctum finder)

For removal of sutures
  1 pair iris scissors
  1 pair suture forceps
  8 swabs
  1 eye pad

Additional packs
  (a) 2 pairs artery forceps ⎫ for suturing of wounds
  (b) 1 pair sinus forceps   ⎭
  (c) 1 pair corneal suture forceps; for removal of corneal sutures
  (d) 1 pair conjunctival scissors; for cutting eye-lashes
  (e) 1 speculum with lash guards
  (f) 1 pair silver wire lid retractors; for examination of babies

The problem of assessing the number of sets required obviously depends on the frequency of re-sterilization as well as on the number of treatments done. Some economy in numbers of instruments can be made by not including too much in every pack but keeping separate instruments for addition as required; for example, speculae packed individually instead of including one in each setting for removal of sutures.

Instruments for ward use would include sets for removal of sutures, syringing of lacrimal sacs, carbolizing corneal ulcers, and scissors for cutting eyelashes.

Eye Dressings

SPECIAL THEATRE REQUIREMENTS

FACE MASKS

These are used for operations in which sutures would lie on the face unless it was protected. They are used for all operations by some surgeons.

Masks can be made of soft muslin; a convenient size is a 16-inch square of double thickness muslin with a circular hole, 2 inches in diameter in the centre.

A simple and effective mask is provided by a 5-inch square of muslin in which the surgeon cuts a central slit and tucks the upper and lower edges under the guards of the speculum: the muslin is discarded after use.

TOWELS

A convenient size for theatre towels is 40 by 24 inches. If two towels are taken and placed on the pillow, the upper one will be wrapped round the head to cover the hair. A specially designed towel, with an appropriate hole, is then used to cover the chest, neck and face leaving the eye for operation conveniently exposed.

2

FIRST AID TO THE EYE

It is no part of a nurse's work to treat eye conditions, but accidents to the eye require the earliest possible treatment owing to the risk to the sight. Pain may make it very difficult to examine an eye without the help of anaesthetic drops and a nurse may only be able to advise the patient to go straight to the doctor: it is always better to go to his surgery rather than to send for him as he will have his special equipment at hand. There are, however, a number of minor injuries for which a nurse can render valuable first aid.

FOREIGN BODIES

Patients are disproportionately grateful for the relief gained from the removal of a foreign body from under the lid.

Method of examination and removal of Foreign Bodies. A good light is essential and the patient's head should be supported as comfortably as circumstances allow. (If the patient is at home, an arm-chair makes a convenient head rest.) In hospital a damp swab stick is used for removal of the foreign body, but if necessary it can be improvised by a match or pencil and for a swab the patient can be asked to lick a corner of his own handkerchief.

The lower fornix and eyeball are first examined: flies often lodge in the inner canthus and can be removed with the tip of a damp swab.

Foreign bodies on the cornea can usually be seen but may need magnification: a nurse should not attempt their removal, but should send the patient to a doctor as soon as possible as they make the eye inflamed and might lead to an ulcer if left.

The upper lid should then be everted (see page 40): a sub-tarsal foreign body is one of the most common and is usually very easily removed with a swab. It is possible for more than one to be present or the piece to break up when touched and therefore a thorough look should be taken when the lid is everted. It is convincing to the patient if he is shown the foreign body on the swab although he will be amazed at how small it is. Immediate relief is the rule and if the patient is still uncomfortable after a few minutes it may indicate that the foreign body scratched the cornea and that is now causing pain. This can be decided by staining the eye with fluorescein and examining for the typical green stain, but a nurse will not have these facilities, and in any case the treatment of a corneal abrasion is work for a doctor.

The following is a simple way of trying to remove a suspected foreign body from under the upper lid. Get the patient to look downwards and draw down the upper lid by the lashes; the patient is then asked to look up and it is hoped that the lashes of the lower lid will have brushed the inner surface of the upper one and in this way have removed the foreign body.

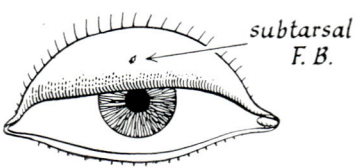

SUB-TARSAL FOREIGN BODY

It cannot be stressed too strongly that unless a foreign body is seen and removed, the patient should not be reassured; it is very easy to find a lash which has probably been put in in the effort of everting the lid and this is seldom the cause of the discomfort. Early conjunctivitis feels like 'grit in the eyes', or there may be a minute corneal foreign body; if the discomfort does not pass off in a few hours medical advice should be sought.

An eye pad is best improvised by a clean soft handkerchief folded in a square over the closed eye and tied firmly with a large handkerchief or wide bandage.

First Aid

LIQUIDS SPLASHED IN THE EYE

A variety of liquids can be splashed or squirted into the eye: for a first-aid measure in the home it is wiser to wash the eye immediately as thoroughly as possible with tap water, before searching for an antidote. Afterwards an alkaline lotion can be made with bicarbonate of soda, one teaspoonful to half a pint of water, or an acid one with boracic powder in the same quantities. Saline, from salt and water, is more soothing than water, but it must be stressed that speed is the important factor in the removal of the irritant and tap water and a clean handkerchief are always at hand.

If the eye hurts and looks red a few drops of paraffin or castor oil will ease it and the patient should be taken to the doctor.

LIME BURNS

Lime in the eye occurs in building work or among children throwing it at each other. It can result in most serious scarring of the cornea, with permanent damage to the sight. The condition is so painful that little effective treatment can be done at home; obvious pieces should be wiped away and perhaps the face held under a tap, but it will be impossible to wash the eyes properly and they should be covered and the patient hurried to the nearest doctor or hospital.

AMMONIA BURNS

The treatment of these is of increasing importance owing to the practice by criminals of spraying ammonia in the faces of their victims when carrying out bank raids or similar assaults. The first-aid treatment is similar to that for lime burns. Hospital treatment is essential as soon as possible and will consist of the treatment for shock, local anaesthetic drops and extremely thorough irrigation with normal saline. Ammonia soaks into the corneal tissues and the eye condition may deteriorate in spite of the most expert treatment. The psychological effect of such an attack is usually serious.

BLACK EYE

This follows a blow, and is due to bruising of the superficial tissues of the lids. The eye is not usually damaged, but the possibility

First Aid

of an orbital fracture should be remembered. If the patient cannot see with the eye medical advice must be sought as there may have been haemorrhage or other injury inside the eyeball.

CUTS OF THE EYELIDS

These are not often serious, but if in the nasal corner the tear passages might be damaged, or if on the upper lid, the levator muscle might be cut.

Even small injuries to the lash margins should be treated by a doctor as there can be very troublesome results from scar deformities, causing the lashes to turn in.

INJURY TO THE EYES

Things may be poked into the eye, e.g. sticks, scissors, pieces of wire, etc. They may cause an abrasion of the cornea or even peforation of the eyeball. The eye should be covered and the patient taken to the doctor at once.

INTRA-OCULAR FOREIGN BODIES

These are often tiny fragments of metal or other material which perforate the eye and remain in it. This occurs most often in men who are using a hammer and chisel or who are employed in work in which fragments of metal are broken off and travel at high speed: numerous safety devices are in use against these industrial accidents A nurse cannot treat the condition, but she should remember the possibility of its occurrence and send the patient for expert advice.

GLOSSARY

Accommodation. The power of the lens to become more convex and so allow near objects to be focused.

Advancement. Operation for squint when the muscle is cut and re-attached nearer to the cornea.

After Cataract. Condition following extra-capsular extraction of lens when the lens capsule is interfering with vision.

Amblyopia (Gr. 'blunt' vision). Used especially when no obvious cause can be found.

Anterior Chamber (A.C.). The space between the cornea in front and the iris and lens behind. It is normally filled with aqueous.

Aphakic Eye. Eye from which the lens has been removed.

Aqueous Humour. A watery fluid, resembling lymph, which is continuously secreted by the ciliary body, circulates in the anterior chamber and drains away at the angle between the cornea and the outer edge of the iris.

Astigmatism. Irregularity of the corneal or lens surface, resulting in the need for spectacles.

Binocular Loupe. A magnifying glass for use with both eyes.

Binocular Vision. Normal vision, in which the individual sees clearly with both eyes the object looked at.

Blepharitis. Inflammation of the lid margins.

Bluestone. Copper sulphate stick.

Bulbar Conjunctivitis. Affecting the conjunctiva covering the eyeball.

Buller's Shield. A watch-glass set in jaconet with the purpose of covering and preventing infection of the second eye from the affected one: not commonly used nowadays.

Glossary

Buphthalmos (Gr. Ox-eye). Glaucoma in a baby when the increased tension causes the eyeball to swell.

Canaliculi. The two passages from the puncta to the lachrymal sac.

Canthus. The angles formed by the junction of the lids; i.e. Inner and Outer.

Capsulotomy. Operation for after-cataract involving the tearing of a hole in the capsule of the lens. 'Needling.'

Carbolization. The painting of a corneal ulcer with 80 per cent carbolic.

Cataract. Opacity of the lens.

Chalazion. Chronic cyst of the meibomian gland near to the lid margin. Meibomian cyst.

Chemosis. Oedema of the conjunctiva.

Cilia. Eye-lashes.

Contact Lens. A spectacle glass made in such a way that it can be worn inside the lids in contact with the cornea.

Cryo Extraction. Method of extraction of the lens using a probe which can be frozen so as to adhere to the lens.

Cryo Therapy. Treatment by cold usually involving the freezing of the tissue concerned.

Cycloplegia. This is the condition of paralysis of the ciliary muscle. It results in the inability of the lens to accommodate for objects near to the eye.

Detachment of Retina. Detachment of the retina from the underlying choroid with consequent loss of vision.

Diplopia. Double vision.

Discission. Operation for soft cataract when the anterior lens capsule is lacerated to allow the lens substance to be absorbed.

Drainage angle. The portion of the anterior chamber where the corneo-scleral junction, the iris and the corneo-scleral trabecular tissue meet. The term is frequently used in connection with glaucoma as the drainage of aqueous takes place in this region.

Ectropion. Turning out of the lid.

Entropion. Turning in of the lid.

Enucleation. Removal of eye.

Epilation. Drawing out of eye-lashes.

Epiphora. Overflow of tears on to the cheek.

Glossary

Evisceration. Removal of the eye by scooping the contents out of the sclera and thus avoiding cutting the optic nerve.

Exenteration of Orbit. Removal of all the soft tissues in the orbit

Exophthalmos. Condition of protrusion of the eye: it is usual to use this term when both eyes are involved, e.g. exophthalmic goitre.

Extraction of Lens. Operation for removal of the lens.

Extra-capsular Extraction. Operation for cataract in which the lens capsule is left.

Fornix. Cul-de-sac where the conjunctiva covering the eyeball is reflected upon the eyelid.

Fundus (L. 'the bottom'). The interior of the eye which can be seen with an ophthalmoscope.

Glaucoma. Increase of tension within the eyeball.

Golden Eye Ointment. Yellow mercuric oxide 1 per cent.

Guttae. Drops for instillation into the eye or ear.

Hordeolum. (L. 'little piece of barley'). Stye.

Hypermetropia. Long sight.

Hyphaema. Blood in the anterior chamber.

Hypopyon. Pus in the anterior chamber.

Iridectomy. Removal of part of the iris.

Iridocyclitis. Inflammation of the iris and the ciliary body.

Keratitis. Inflammation of the cornea.

Keratitis Punctata, 'K.P.'. White deposits, occurring in Cyclitis, due to the circulation of this material in the aqueous.

Lachrymal Apparatus. Tear apparatus.

Lamellae. Gelatin discs containing drugs for insertion into the lower fornix.

Limbus. Junction of the cornea with the conjunctiva.

Macula Lutea. The area of most acute vision on the retina.

Meibomian Cyst. Chronic cyst of gland at the edge of the lid.

Miotic. An agent which constricts the pupil.

Mydriatic. An agent which dilates the pupil.

Myopia. Short sight.

Needling. Capsulotomy: the capsule of the lens is torn with a special needle.

Nystagmus (Gr. to nod.). Involuntary rapid oscillation of the eyeball.

Glossary

Oculentum. Eye ointment.

Ophthalmia Neonatorum. Inflamation of the eyes of the newborn; if occurring under twenty-one days it is a notifiable disease.

Orthoptics. Special exercises to encourage binocular vision.

Palpebral Conjunctiva. Conjunctiva lining the eyelids.

Panophthalmitis. Inflammation involving the whole eyeball.

Paracentesis. Tapping of the anterior chamber.

Perimeter. An instrument for measuring the extent of the visual field.

Photophobia. Fear of light.

Presbyopia. Reduced power of accommodation due to advancing age.

Proptosis. Protusion of the eyeball.

Ptosis. Drooping of the upper lid.

Refraction. The testing of vision to estimate the degree of refractive error, e.g. astigmatism.

Strabismus (Gr. 'to turn'). Squint.

Symblepharon. Adhesions of the lids to the eyeball.

Synechia. Adhesion of the iris to the lens behind, or to the cornea in front.

Tarsorrhaphy. Suturing together of the lid margins over the eyeball.

Tenotomy. Operation for squint involving the division or weakening of the fibres of a muscle.

Trachoma. A serious type of granular conjunctivitis.

Trephining. Operation for glaucoma in which a small disc is removed at the cornea-scleral margin for artificial drainage of aqueous.

Trichiasis. Condition of the eye-lashes so that they are directed backwards and rub against the cornea.

Uveitis. Inflammation of the pigmented layer of the eye comprising the iris, ciliary body and choroid.

Visual Acuity. Acuteness or clearness of vision.

Visual Field. Area within which objects may be seen.

Vitreous. A clear transparent mass of gelatinous consistency which fills the eyeball behind the lens.

INDEX

Abscission of iris prolapse, 152
Accommodation, 217
Acuity of vision, 22
Advancement, 181, 217
After cataract, 153, 217
Amblyopia, 217
Ammonia burns, 215
Anaesthetic, local, 52
Anterior chamber, 35, 217
Antiseptic drops, 53
Aphakia, 217
Applications to conjunctiva, 77
Aqueous humour, 35, 217
Artificial eye, 186
Astigmatism, 217
Atropine irritation, 50

Bacteriological culture, 85
Bandaging, 107
Bathing, cold, 74
 ,, hot, 69
Binocular loupe, 34
Bjerrum Screen, 29
Black eye, 120, 215
Blepharitis, 39, 55, 217
Bluestone, 217
Bulbar conjunctiva, 217
Buller's shield, 217
Buphthalmos, 218
Burns, injuries caused by, 120, 121

Canaliculus, 189, 218
Canthus, 218
Capsulectomy, 138
Capsulotomy, 153, 218
Carbolization, 90, 210, 218
Cartella shield, 116
Casualty Department, 118
Cataract, 137, 218
Chalazion, 91, 218
Chemosis, 35, 218
Children, examination of, 22
Cilia, 218
Cold applications, 74
Colour vision, 30
Conjunctival painting, 77
Contact lens, 99, 218
Copper stick, 78
Cornea, 35
Corneal abrasion, 107, 119
Corneal grafting, 159
Corneal foreign body, 89, 210
Cryo extraction, 139, 195, 218
Cryo therapy, 174, 195, 218
Cut eyelids, 216
Cutting of lashes, 74
Cycloplegia, 51, 218
Cyst, meibomian, 91

Dacryocystitis, 188
Dacryocystorhinostomy, 190

INDEX

Dark glasses, 116
Dark room test, 166
Detachment of retina, 173
Diet, 143
Dilator, punctum, 83
Diplopia, 122, 218
Discission, 138, 218
Dressing of eye, post-operative, 145
Dressings, 207
Drops, 42
Drop bottles, 43, 44
Drop bottle stand, 46

'E'-Test, 24, 25
Ectropion, 218
Edridge Green Lantern, 31
Electrolysis, 76
Encircling band operation, 174
Entropion, 79, 218
Enucleation, 184, 218
Epilation, 76, 210, 218
Epiphora, 83, 188, 218
Eversion of lids, 39, 40, 214
Evisceration, 186, 219
Examination of eye, 19
Excision of eyeball, 184
Exenteration of orbit, 186, 219
Exophthalmos, 219
Expression of lachrymal sac, 80
Extraction of lens, 138, 219
Eye bath, 68
,, pads, 209
,, shades, 111, 115, 117
,, swabs, 207, 208

Feeding of patients, 143
Field of vision, 26
First aid, 213
Fluorescein, 54
Foreign body, corneal, 89, 119, 213
,, ,, intra-ocular, 89, 119, 216
,, ,, subtarsal, 89, 119, 214

Fornix, 219
Fundus, 219

Glass rod, 56
Glaucoma, 121, 162, 219
Gonioscopy, 164
Graefe knife, 138
Guttae, 49, 219

Hordeolun, 219
Hot bathing, 69
,, fomentation, 72
,, pad, 72
Hypermetropia, 219
Hyphaema, 36, 151, 219
Hypopyon, 36, 219

Iced bathing, 74
Incision and curettage of meibomian cyst, 91, 210
Injection, subconjunctival, 94
,, retrobulbar, 95
Injuries to eyeball, 172, 216
Insensitive eye, 81
Inspection lamp, 19
Instillation of drops, 42, 45
Instruments, 38, 199, 201, 209
Insufflation, 79
Intra-ocular lenses, 157
,, foreign body, 119, 216
Iridectomy, 219
Iridocyclitis, 219
Iris, observation of, 3
,, prolapse, 151
Iritis, post-operative, 151
Irrigation, 59
,, of anterior chamber, 202
Ishihara Colour Test, 31

Keratitis, 219
Keratome, 138
Keratoplasty, 159
Knives, care of, 199

INDEX

Lachrymal apparatus, 189, 219
    ,,   probing, 84, 189
    ,,   syringing, 83, 211
    ,,   sac, expression of, 80
    ,,   ,, , excision of, 190
Lamellae, 79, 219
Lamps, hand, 19, 35
    ,,   theatre, 192
Lid, eversion of, 40
Lid retractor, 89
Lighting in theatre, 192
    ,,   in ward, 131
Limbus, 219
Lime burns, 120, 215
Local anaesthesia, 51
Lotions, 59, 202
Loupes, 34

Macula lutea, 219
Magnet, 195, 196, 197
Massage, 171
Meibomian cyst, 91, 211
Mental confusion, 153
Metricautery, 91
Miotic, 51, 219
Moorfield's bandage, 111
Mydriatic, 50, 219
Mydriatic Test, 166
Myopia, 219

Needles, 138, 202
Needling, 154, 219
Nystagmus, 219

Occlusion, 179
Oculentum, 54, 220
Ointment, application of, 56
Ophthalmia neonatorum, 220
Ophthalmoscopic examination, 20
Orbit, exenteration, 186, 219
Orthoptics, 181, 220
Outpatient Department, 124

Pads, 209

Panophthalmitis, 220
Paracentesis, 220
Perforating wounds, 120, 172
Perimeter, 28, 220
Peripheral field, 28
Phasing, 164
Photocoagulation, 174
Photophobia, 37, 220
Pipettes, 43
Plastic operations, 190
'Plomb' operation, 175
Presbyopia, 220
Probing of lachrymal passages, 84, 189
Prolapse of iris, 151
Proptosis, 220
Provocative glaucoma tests, 165
Ptosis, 190, 220
Punctum, lachrymal, 189
Pupil, irregularities of, 37

Recession, 181
Refraction, 179, 220
Resection, 174, 181
Retina, detachment of, 173
Retrobulbar injection, 95
Rose Bengal, 54

Schiötz Tonometer, 97
Schirmer's Test, 99
Scleral resection, 174
Sclerotomy, 170
Sepsis, post-operative, 152
Sheridan Gardner Test, 25
Sight tests, 22
Silk sutures, 201
Silver nitrate, 77
Slit lamp, 20, 165
Socket, care of, 185
Snellen's test type, 22
Spectacles, 122, 154, 155, 179
Speculum, 88
Spontex, 208
Spud, 90

INDEX

Squint, 178
Staining of cornea, 54
Steam bathing, 70
Sterilizers, 192
Strabismus, 178, 220
Strapping for entropion, 79
Subconjunctival injection, 94
Sutures, 201, 209, 211
    ,,   removal of, 87, 211
Swabbing of eyes, 38
Symblepharon, 58, 173, 184, 220
Sympathetic ophthalmia, 173, 184
Synechia, 220
Syringing of sac, 83, 211

Tarsorrhaphy, 162, 220
Tension, intra-ocular, 96
Testing of knives, 199
Test types, 22, 26
Theatre work, 192

Tissue dispenser, 47
Tonography, 164
Tonometry, 96
Trachoma, 78, 220
Trephines, care of, 200
Trephining, 170, 200
Trial drum, 200
Trichiasis, 161, 220

Ulcer of cornea, 90
Undine, 60
Uveitis, 220

Visual acuity, 22, 220
Visual field, 26, 220
Vitreous, 220

Ward equipment, 131
Water drinking test, 166
Witnessing drops, 49